Lean Behavioral Health

Lean Behavioral Health

THE KINGS COUNTY HOSPITAL STORY

EDITED BY

JOSEPH P. MERLINO, MD, MPA
Director of Psychiatry & Deputy Executive Director
Behavioral Health Services
Kings County Hospital Center
Brooklyn, NY

JOANNA OMI
Senior Vice President/Chief Innovation Officer
Organizational Innovation & Effectiveness
New York City Health & Hospitals Corporation
New York, NY

JILL BOWEN, PhD
Sr. Associate Executive Director/Chief of Staff
Behavioral Health Services
Kings County Hospital Center
Brooklyn, NY

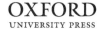

OXFORD
UNIVERSITY PRESS

OXFORD
UNIVERSITY PRESS

Oxford University Press is a department of the University of Oxford.
It furthers the University's objective of excellence in research, scholarship,
and education by publishing worldwide.

Oxford   New York
Auckland   Cape Town   Dar es Salaam   Hong Kong   Karachi
Kuala Lumpur   Madrid   Melbourne   Mexico City   Nairobi
New Delhi   Shanghai   Taipei   Toronto

With offices in
Argentina   Austria   Brazil   Chile   Czech Republic   France   Greece
Guatemala   Hungary   Italy   Japan   Poland   Portugal   Singapore
South Korea   Switzerland   Thailand   Turkey   Ukraine   Vietnam

Oxford is a registered trademark of Oxford University Press
in the UK and certain other countries.

Published in the United States of America by
Oxford University Press
198 Madison Avenue, New York, NY 10016

Library of Congress Cataloging-in-Publication Data
Lean behavioral health : the Kings County Hospital story / edited by Joseph P. Merlino,
Joanna Omi, Jill Bowen.
     p.; cm.
Includes index.
ISBN 978–0–19–998952–2 (alk. paper)
I. Merlino, Joseph P., editor of compilation.   II. Omi, Joanna, editor of compilation.
III. Bowen, Jill, editor of compilation.
[DNLM: 1. Kings County Hospital (Kings County, N.Y.)   2. Psychiatric Department,
Hospital—organization & administration—New York.   3. Hospitals, Municipal—organization &
administration—New York.   4. Mental Health Services—organization & administration—New York.
5. Organizational Culture—New York. WM 28 AN6]
RC445.N7 L43 2014
362.2′10974723—dc23   2013025970

This material is not intended to be, and should not be considered, a substitute for medical or other professional
advice. Treatment for the conditions described in this material is highly dependent on the individual circumstances. And, while this material is designed to offer accurate information with respect to the subject matter
covered and to be current as of the time it was written, research and knowledge about medical and health issues
is constantly evolving and dose schedules for medications are being revised continually, with new side effects
recognized and accounted for regularly. Readers must therefore always check the product information and
clinical procedures with the most up-to-date published product information and data sheets provided by the
manufacturers and the most recent codes of conduct and safety regulation. The publisher and the authors make
no representations or warranties to readers, express or implied, as to the accuracy or completeness of this material. Without limiting the foregoing, the publisher and the authors make no representations or warranties as to
the accuracy or efficacy of the drug dosages mentioned in the material. The authors and the publisher do not
accept, and expressly disclaim, any responsibility for any liability, loss or risk that may be claimed or incurred as
a consequence of the use and/or application of any of the contents of this material.

9 8 7 6 5 4 3 2 1
Printed in the United States of America
on acid-free paper

This book is dedicated to the HHC community—the 37,000 problem solvers who represent the future of HHC

The Editors wish to thank the many people whose work and compassion are represented in this book. We are indebted to colleagues who provided guidance and counsel throughout the writing of this book. Our journey has been guided by many who have traveled this road before us, including leaders and sensei from Simpler North America and our friends and mentors who have shared what they have accomplished so that we may learn from their experience.

On a personal note, the Editors would like to acknowledge Ron, (JPM); Grant, Yoshi, Colin and Julie (JO); Rich, Jeffrey, and Ian (JB). Thank you for your unending support.

Contents

Preface

When the New York City Health and Hospitals Corporation (HHC) began its lean journey in late 2007, we were hopeful, excited, expectant, and ... sinfully ignorant. We knew that others in health care—notably Denver Health, ThedaCare, and Virginia Mason—had pioneered the application of lean principles, values, and practices in health care to extraordinary results. But we really had little understanding of what we would be getting into. We did have confidence in our ability to make change, and as we describe in Chapter 1, we recognized the need for deep, transformative action that could help us break through the entrenched resistance to change that characterized our large, municipal bureaucracy and that too frequently stymied our attempts to innovate. We were also concerned that, with all of the tools in our armamentarium (from years of adopting the health care improvement method of the moment), we had yet to come close to solving the challenges of spread and sustainment. To do so, and to take HHC to greater heights of clinical quality, patient safety, and operational efficiency, we would have to behave and perform differently than we had in the past. We didn't sign up for lean lightly—we promised our board of directors substantial change and they responded with a not insubstantial budgetary approval to jump-start the effort.

Health care in the United States is being turned on its head. The Centers for Medicaid and Medicare (CMS) is moving toward denial of payments for "never events" and certain avoidable patient stays and readmissions. Hospital systems are forming partnerships on the road to becoming Accountable Care Organizations, investing in IT to obtain Meaningful Use payments, and crafting Patient Centered Medical Homes and Health Homes as incipient payment reform begins to reverse incentives to provide ever more inpatient care and other high-cost services. With the 2012 Supreme Court rejection of challenges posed to key provisions of the Patient Protection and Affordable Care Act, health care as we have known and provided it will never be the same. Some states have launched their own bold payment reform initiatives, and together with fast evolving federal reforms, these policy initiatives represent an unprecedented paradigm shift and a platform afire.

Lean in hospitals is still a relatively new phenomenon. We are indebted to those health care pioneers who saw the hope of lean, sought to learn about it, explored ways to adopt it in a new setting, and shared their stories with us. In particular, Dr. Patricia Gabow, CEO of Denver Health until 2012, gave generously of her time and expertise and helped inspire and launch our journey. The early lean pioneers in health care were not so fortunate and had to look to manufacturing to understand what lean looked like and what its application could do for an organization. From a snow-blowing and lawn mower manufacturer (Thedacare sought guidance from Ariens), to a builder of jets (Virginia Mason established a relationship with Boeing), and across many industries (Denver Health created an advisory board with Ritz-Carlton and FedEx representatives), manufacturers and companies from many other sectors have much to teach us. After our initial doubt ("Patients aren't widgets!"), we have been eager to listen and learn.

In 2013, with 6 years of lean behind us, HHC's lean effort is still in in its infancy. We have a long, long road ahead of us but hope that with this book, others may stand on our shoulders to achieve even greater results as we collectively redefine health care in the United States. Although we are implementing lean across our entire, vast public hospital system, this book focuses on what we have experienced and learned in one area—behavioral health—and, for the most part, in one hospital—Kings County Hospital Center. We believe we have only uncovered the first epithelial layer of what lean can offer us, and it has been a hard, enlightening and immensely satisfying journey. The rewards in staff engagement and empowerment, in the degree to which we have been able to bring value to patients, and, not the least, the reduction of waste and generation of significant revenue, have been tremendous.

This book is not intended to be an authoritative treatise on lean. We do not profess to be experts and are still quite early in our journey. However, we know that many in health care share our conviction that we need a massive shift in the paradigm of modern health care—deep, systemic change in how we think of our work, the people we do it for, and the people who do it. Lean is helping us to see through fresh eyes and to reach deep inside ourselves for reserves of innovation, patience and purposeful compassion long depressed by crisis management and an abundance of waste. If you, like us, aspire to render ever better, more affordable care to patients, we hope you find value in our story.

With humility and great pride,

Alan Aviles
President and Chief Executive Officer
New York City Health and Hospitals Corporation
January 2013

About the Editors

Joseph P. Merlino is the chief executive for behavioral health services and Director of Psychiatry at Kings County Hospital Center, where he leads the transformation efforts of one of the largest public hospitals in New York. Previously he was Director of Psychiatry at Queens Hospital Center. He is also Professor of Psychiatry at the State University of New York — Downstate Medical College and Adjunct Professor of Psychiatry and Behavioral Sciences at New York Medical College. He received a Master's Degree in Public Administration from Baruch College, City University of New York. Dr. Merlino is on the Board of Directors for the Group for the Advancement of Psychiatry where he chairs the Committee on Administration and Leadership. Dr. Merlino is a Distinguished Fellow of the American Psychiatric Association and a Fellow of the American College of Psychiatrists. He is a past president of the American Academy of Psychoanalysis and Dynamic Psychiatry.

Joanna Omi is chief innovation officer and senior vice president for organizational innovation and effectiveness at the New York City Health and Hospitals Corporation (HHC). Ms. Omi provides leadership and operational guidance to Breakthrough, the HHC Enterprise-wide Improvement System. She is responsible for the development and adoption of lean throughout HHC's healthcare facilities and corporate offices. Prior to her current position, Ms. Omi was HHC's Senior Assistant Vice President for Corporate Planning and HIV Services. In this capacity, she led the Corporation's planning efforts and managed special projects, including the Corporate Ambulatory Care Restructuring Initiative, the Community Health Care Demonstration Project, HIV/AIDS programs and development of the first federally qualified health center on Staten Island. Previously, Ms. Omi was Executive Director of the New York City HIV Health and Human Services Planning Council, served as Senior Policy Analyst for Budget and Legislation in the Mayor's Office on Health Policy, and directed HIV/AIDS and prenatal programs in the Bay Area.

Jill Bowen is the senior associate executive director and chief of staff for Behavioral Health Services at Kings County Hospital Center. Trained as a clinical psychologist, she received her master's degree and doctoral degree in clinical psychology at the Derner Institute for Advanced Psychological Studies/Adelphi University. Her work has included direct care as a member of an interdisciplinary acute care clinical team and supervisory work in clinical and forensic psychology. She was the Deputy Director and unit chief of the Forensic Psychiatry Service at Kings County Hospital Center before moving on to work as a senior administrator within Behavioral Health, focusing on strategic planning and process improvement. She has worked at Kings County Hospital Center for the past 26 years and has played a significant role in the transformation of the services provided in the Behavioral Health department across the continuum of care.

Contributors

Akinola Adebisi, MD
Medical Director Adult Outpatient
Behavior Health Services
Kings County Hospital Center
Brooklyn, NY

Renuka Ananthamoorthy, MD
Chief of Service
Behavioral Health Services
Kings County Hospital
CenterBrooklyn, NY

Kristen Baumann, PhD
Lean/Breakthrough Deployment
    Officer
Metropolitan Hospital Center
New York, NY

Robert Berding, Esq., LMHC, CRC
Associate Executive Director,
    Regulatory Compliance/Risk
    Management
Patient Safety Officer
Kings County Hospital Center
Brooklyn, NY

Jill Bowen, PhD
Sr. Associate Executive
    Director/Chief of Staff
Behavioral Health Services
Kings County Hospital Center
Brooklyn, NY

Regine Bruny-Olawaiye, MD/MBA
Director of Comprehensive Psychiatric
    Emergency Program
Behavioral Health Services
Kings County Hospital Center
Brooklyn, NY

Olga Deshchenko
Assistant Director
Internal Communications Group
New York City Health and Hospitals
    Corporation
New York, NY

Lancelot Deygoo, MSCE
Behavioral Health Finance
Behavioral Health Services
Kings County Hospital Center
Brooklyn, NY

Richard J. Freeman
Associate Executive Director
Behavioral Health
Metropolitan Hospital Center
New York, NY

Lora Giacomoni, RN, MSN
Sr. Associate Director, Quality &
    Compliance
Behavioral Health Services
Kings County Hospital Center
Brooklyn, NY

Todd Hixson, MBA
Associate Executive Director, Acute
    and Critical Care
Metropolitan Hospital Center
New York, NY

Antonio D. Martin
Executive Vice President/Chief
    Operating Officer
New York City Health & Hospitals
    Corporation
New York, NY

Joseph P. Merlino, MD, MPA
Director of Psychiatry & Deputy
    Executive Director
Behavioral Health Services
Kings County Hospital Center
Brooklyn, NY

Roumen N. Nikolov, MD
Associate Chief of Service
Behavior Health Services
Kings County Hospital Center
Brooklyn, NY

Joanna Omi
Senior Vice President/Chief
    Innovation Officer
Organizational Innovation &
    Effectiveness
New York City Health & Hospitals
    Corporation
New York, NY

Linda Paradiso, RN, MSN, NEA-BC
Associate Executive Director,
    BH Nursing
Behavioral Health Services
Kings County Hospital Center
Brooklyn, NY

Claire Patterson, MS, RD
Breakthrough Deployment Officer
Kings County Hospital Center
Brooklyn, NY

Janine Perazzo, LCSW
Behavioral Health Director of Social Work
Kings County Hospital Center
Brooklyn, NY

George Proctor
Network Senior Vice President/
    Executive Director
North Central Brooklyn Health
    Network
Woodhull Medical & Mental
    Health Center
Brooklyn, NY

Ameer Robertson, Esq.
Lean/Breakthrough Deployment Officer
Generations Plus Network Diagnostic &
    Treatment Centers (D&TCs)
New York City Health & Hospitals
    Corporation (HHC)

Bruce Smith
Senior Consultant
Simpler North America
Pittsburgh, PA

Joyce B. Wale, LCSW
Senior Assistant Vice President
Office of Behavioral Health
New York City Health & Hospitals
    Corporation
New York, NY

Roslyn S. Weinstein, MEd
Senior Assistant Vice President,
    Operations
New York City Health & Hospitals
    Corporation
New York, NY

Marlene Zurack
Senior Vice President/Chief Financial
    Officer
New York City Health & Hospitals
    Corporation
New York, NY

Glossary of Lean Terms

Term	Definition	Use
6S	Used for improving organization of the workplace, the name comes from the six steps required to implement and the words (each starting with S) used to describe each step: sort, straighten, scrub, safety, standardize, and sustain	Create a safe, efficient, and organized work area
A3 thinking	Forces consensus building; unifies culture around a simple systematic, methodology; becomes also a communication tool that follows a logical narrative; and builds over years as organization learning; A3 = metric nomenclature for a paper size equal to 11" x 17"	Strategy, Planning, VSA, RIE, problem solving
Andon	A device, or signal, that calls attention to defects, equipment abnormalities, or other problems or reports the status and needs of a system typically but not always by means of *lights*—red light for failure mode, amber light to show marginal performance, and a green light for normal operation mode	Visual management tool
Bottleneck	The place in the value stream that negatively affects throughput/restricts flow; as a resource capacity limitation, a bottleneck will not allow a system to meet the demand of the customer	Constraint or flow stopper

Term	Definition	Use
Catchball	The process of selecting strategies to meet an objective at any level then getting managers and their teams to engage in dialogue to reach agreement on strategies to achieve their goals	Collaborative goal setting
Gemba	Japanese word of which the literal translation is "the real place"; used to describe the work unit where value is created, where work is done	Go and see the work
Fishbone diagram	Also called an Ishikawa diagram, this tool is a schematic problem-solving tool that resembles a fish skeleton, with a main spine ending in a head in which a problem statement is placed, and branches (bones) drawn at a slant off the spine that typically represent categories (people, method, machine, materials, environment); used as a cause-and-effect diagram, where the spine denotes an effect and the branches are cause factors	Establish direct and root causes of the effect or problem
Five whys	Practice of asking "why" five times when a problem is encountered; repeated questioning helps identify the root cause of a problem so that effective countermeasures can be developed and implemented	Determine root causes of problems
Flow	The progressive achievement of tasks and/or information as it proceeds along the value stream, flow challenges us to reorganize the value stream to be continuous...."one by one, nonstop"	Describes efficient, "least waste" movement
Flow cell	A logical, efficient, and usually physically self-contained arrangement of supplies, equipment, and personnel to complete a service sequence; a flow cell enables visual management, simple flow, standard work, pull, 6S, transparency, and tight connections	Usually a series of linked cells, provides the environment in which the "least waste" way can be accomplished

Term	Definition	Use
Milk run	The routing of a supply or delivery to make multiple, repeating pickups or drop-offs at different locations; milk runs are made by suppliers or cooperating groups of suppliers who make frequent, small deliveries to customers who practice just-in-time delivery and maintain a low inventory	Used in the creation of products with multiple-piece parts to maintain low inventory while reliably meeting customer demand
Pareto graph	A vertical bar graph in which data is represented in descending order of frequency, ordered from left to right, to ascertain relative and cumulative contribution to a problem; a graphic demonstration of the Pareto Principle suggests that the significant items in a given group normally constitute a relatively small portion of the items in the total group. Conversely, a majority of the items will be relatively minor in significance (i.e., the 80/20 rule)	Trend analysis for root cause problem solving "vital few vs. the trivial many"
Perfection	Never-ending pursuit of the complete elimination of non-value-adding waste so that all activities along a value stream create value; perfection challenges us to also create compelling quality ("defect free") while also reducing cost ("lowest cost")	Lean principle
Point of use	The condition in which all supplies are within arm's reach and positioned in the sequence in which they are used to prevent extra reaching, lifting, straining, turning, and twisting	Supplies at where the work is completed
Pull	Deliver value to customers on demand; pull challenges us to only respond "on demand" to our downstream customers	Lean principle

Term	Definition	Use
Pull system/ Kanban	Visual process that connects customers to their suppliers; conveys critical information to ensure controls of the right item or response in the necessary quantity and the necessary time; replenishes the consumption of items flowing in a process	Signal that material is required
Mistake proof/ Poka-Yoke	"Innocent mistake-proofing"; an improvement technique that uses a device or procedure, also called a *poka-yoke*, to prevent defects or equipment malfunction during order-taking or manufacture	Describes proactive error prevention
RIE/Kaizen	Rapid improvement event (RIE) is a 4.5-day process utilizing a team-based methodology to apply the lean tools for seeing waste and making rapid improvement during the event	4.5-day process for implementing change
Standard work	An agreed-upon set of work procedures that effectively combines people, materials, and machines to maintain quality, efficiency, safety, and predictability; work is described precisely in terms of cycle time, work in process, sequence, takt time, layout, and the inventory needed to conduct the activity	Written description of the "best known way" to do work
Standards	Rules or examples that provide clear expectations	Standards let us see abnormalities
TPOC	Transformation Plan of Care = the plan for transforming a business; documented using an A3, this is the executive level road map for a defined period of time	Creating vision and alignment over the course of the transformation
Takt time	The rate at which product must be turned out to satisfy market demand. It is determined by dividing the available production time by the rate of customer demand	Nontraditional use: meeting time –that is, start time 10 a.m., takt 1 hour

Lean term	Definition	Use
Value	When a product or service has been perceived or appraised to fulfill a need or desire—*as defined by the customer*—the product or service may be said to have value or worth. Components of value may include quality, utility, functionality, capacity, aesthetics, timeliness or availability, price, etc.	Lean principle "Does our customer want to pay for this?"
Value stream	All the activities (both value-added and non-value-added) required within an organization to deliver a specific service; "everything that goes into" creating and delivering the "value" to the end customer	Lean principle
Value stream analysis	The identification of all the specific activities occurring along the value stream, represented pictorially in a value stream map; see waste, unevenness, and overburden, size the opportunity, share a vision, communicate visually, permission to change, predict results	"See" and develop a value stream vision/future state road map
Vertical value stream mapping	Enables "one-off" activities to flow without waste; used for improving "non-recurring" processes; works for highly complex processes; a key enabler for multidisciplinary teams	Lean project management
Visual management	Visually controlled processes in the workplace, where anyone in the area should have a good idea about the who, what, where, when, why, and how of activities and equipment within minutes or seconds	At a glance rule
Voice of the customer	The desires and expectations of the customer, which are of primary importance in the development of new products, services, and the daily conduct of the business	Listening to and acting on customer feedback

Lean term	Definition	Use
Waste/Muda	Any operation or activity that takes time and resources but does not add value to the product or service sold to the customer	Non-value-added work
Water Strider or Water Spider/ Mizusumashi	Someone who moves quickly and efficiently from place to place to collect and deliver material/supplies to the primary members of a flow cell; move as much of the non-value-added work away from the primary member as possible and "centralize" it on the water spider	Improving the delivery of the value through improved efficiency of the primary worker
5 Lean Principles	Value Value stream Flow Pull Perfection	Steps to guide lean implementation
6S	Sort Straighten Scrub Safety Standardize Sustain	Tool
8 Wastes	Defects Overproduction Waiting Not best use of talent Transportation Inventory Motion Extra processing "Acronym: D.O.W.N.T.I.M.E."	Learning to see waste in a process

Acronym	Description	Use
A3	Metric size of paper = 11" x 17"—9 boxes designed to tell the event story	Tool
RIE	Rapid improvement event	Tool
POU	Point of use	Tool
TPOC	Transformation plan of care	A3 type
TPS	Toyota production system	Philosophy
VOC	Voice of customer	Tool
VSA	Value stream analysis	Tool

Japanese	English
Gemba	The place where the work is done
Kaizen	Rapid improvement event (RIE)
Kanban	Pull system
Mizusumashi	Water strider or water spider
Muda	Waste
Poka-yoke	Mistake or error proof

1

Why Lean in Health Care—People Aren't Cars

JOANNA OMI, BRUCE SMITH, AND AMEER ROBERTSON

The New York City Health and Hospitals Corporation (HHC) is the largest municipal health care system in the country. Our history includes many firsts—the oldest continuously operating hospital in the United States, the first ambulance, the first hospital wards for mental health and alcoholism and many innovations in medicine and public health dating back to the early 1700s. With an operating budget of $6.7 billion, HHC provides medical, mental health and substance abuse services through 11 acute care hospitals, 4 skilled nursing facilities, 6 large diagnostic and treatment facilities, a health maintenance organization (the 420,000-member health plan, MetroPlus), and a home care agency. Serving 1.4 million New Yorkers annually, more than 475,000 of whom are uninsured, HHC operates 7,626 beds and provides almost 5 million outpatient visits, 1.1 million emergency room visits, and more than 250,000 admissions a year. HHC is humbled to have been recognized by the National Quality Forum, the National Association of Public Hospitals and Health Systems, the Institute for Healthcare Improvement, and The Joint Commission for its contributions to patient safety, innovation, and community service.

No health care organization is immune from the turmoil and uncertainty that defines health care in the United States today. Significant reductions in Medicare and Medicaid spending, the imposition of quality standards that define federal government payments, requirements that health care organizations coordinate patient care across systems, and ever more limiting coverage by traditional health insurers together mandate enormous change on the part of all care providers and institutions. Some of us have turned to lean, the term coined by a group of researchers from the Massachusetts Institute of Technology to capture the principles and tools of the Toyota Production System (TPS) as a means of addressing the significant demands imposed by our constantly changing environment.[1]

What Is Lean?

Over time, practitioners have defined lean in different ways. However, at its most pure, lean is what Toyota created and applied through the Toyota Way and the related Toyota Production System (TPS). Jeffrey K. Liker, a leading authority on Toyota, describes the Toyota Way as articulating the foundational principles of the Toyota culture, and it is this foundation upon which TPS, the operating system that enables the company to consistently and reliably build a variety of high-quality cars while maintaining a strong financial position, is built.[2] Toyota has been known as the lean authority for more than 50 years and the most current lean improvement philosophies and approaches are constructed using TPS as a foundation. TPS is based on the core principles of respect for people, society, and customers and continuous improvement. Respect is not just a word at Toyota; it is actively practiced every day by engaging their people and customers to continuously improve all of their core product lines and processes. It is often touted that Toyota is in the business of building people first and exceptional cars second.

TPS is defined as a series of processes by James Womack and Daniel Jones in *Lean Thinking*. These are:

- defining value (from the customer's perspective);
- defining the value stream (the set of all steps required to produce a product or service);
- ensuring that the product or service or its component parts or actions flow smoothly across the value stream without interruption; and
- responding to "pull" (each step in the value stream takes place only in response to a downstream trigger, eliminating excess inventory and wasted movement), working toward excellence or zero defects.

From the Factory to Health Care

Lean management systems modeled after TPS have been successfully implemented in the manufacturing industry for more than three decades. One such example occurred from 1992 to 1999 at HON Company (now HNI Corporation), located in Iowa. HON Company is a manufacturer of office furniture products. This transformation was led by George Koenigsaecker, a proven executive leader and an early adopter of lean. Koenigsaecker and his courageous staff embarked on their lean journey and achieved very impressive results. On average, the following results were achieved each year from 1992 to 1999: reduced employee accident rate by 20%; reduced errors and customer complaint rates by 20%; reduced lead times by 50%; and increased enterprise productivity by 15%. These results positioned HON from being number 5 in their industry to number 2 (growing sales just under three times through "organic" growth). Koenigsaecker stated, "This is not a pace of improvement that I would recommend to someone just starting out on their lean journey, as it was challenging, to say the least." It is especially impressive that HON (HNI) is still engaged with the lean transformation efforts started more than 20 years ago.[3]

In the spirit of complete transparency, for every HON Company, there are also a fair number of manufacturing organizations that have attempted to implement lean and have failed. The most common theme for failure seems to revolve around the fact that lean implementations are not for the faint of heart. Translated, organizations fail to realize that lean is a journey and cannot be effectively implemented and sustained across the enterprise in a short period of time, such as 1 to 3 years. In fact, according to the Industry Week/MPI Census of Manufacturers, almost 70% of manufacturing plants in the United States were utilizing lean at the time of a 2007 survey; the popularity of lean among the survey group was twice that of Total Quality Management, the next most commonly applied improvement method. Still, only 2% of survey respondents reported successfully meeting objectives, and only 24% secured results of significance using lean.[4] Although similar data are not known to be available in the health care sector, a growing number of studies include observations of health care organizations among those made of businesses with deeper roots in continuous improvement, such as manufacturing, aerospace, and business.

Most organizations do not have the patience to allow a lean culture to evolve over time, to enable the slow bake that can produce world-class results. Studies of performance improvement and organizational culture consistently identify a short list of common failure modes and their corollary elements of success. Steven Spear of the Massachusetts Institute of Technology cites four "capabilities of high-velocity organizations": (1) specifying design to capture existing knowledge and building in tests to reveal problems; (2) swarming and solving problems to build new knowledge; (3) sharing new knowledge throughout the organization; and (4) leading by developing the first three capabilities.[5] Abrahamson (2000), recognizing the toll change fatigue plays on the psyche and stamina of an organization, emphasizes four operating guidelines that are exemplified by companies that successfully changed over time (IBM, American Express, and GE). These companies reward shameless borrowing, appreciate institutional memory (a "chief memory officer" can help the company avoid making the same old mistakes), tinker and kludge—experiment— internally before searching for solutions externally, and hire generalists (people who can bring fresh, unbiased eyes to problem solving).[6]

Liker and Rother evaluated their own earlier work and concluded that long-lasting change requires much more than mastery of tools. Rather, organizations that expect, achieve, and sustain excellence learn not just how to apply solutions but how to utilize tools to create a constant state of learning and improving.[7] Chakravorty supports the often-cited dictum that "extended involvement" of an improvement expert is a success factor for process improvement programs. He described such experts as necessary "if teams are to remain motivated, continue learning and maintain early gains." So important are these teachers/experts that it was found to be just as successful to have one assigned *part-time* to several teams over 1 to 2 years while training managers to eventually take over the "expert role."[8]

Sensei, a Japanese word meaning "teacher" and often used to describe lean experts, describes a mode of work that tends to be different from traditional consultancies. Sensei will encourage clients to learn by doing (rather than doing for clients) and by asking provocative questions. If you hire a sensei and expect to be told what to do, you will be very disappointed. The process of transferring knowledge and skill development from sensei to client is intense and expectations are high. You will not be receiving a report with fancy graphs detailing how to get your business back on track. Most likely your sensei is going to take you on a "field trip" of your own work place—your first *gemba* walk.[9]

The lean sensei teaches and guides the organization on their path to lean implementation and ultimately business transformation. Often the sensei is an external consultant to the organization, bringing in specialized skills. A lean journey does not require the use of a sensei, but having one can help to jump-start the initial learning phase and support an accelerated pace, both of which facilitate workforce engagement and shorten the time between theory and successful application. One of the main ways a sensei guides and teaches organizations is through gemba walks and teaching what is not lean about processes in value streams. Sensei are instrumental in helping organizations get lean implementation off the ground and serve as objective parties ensuring lean initiatives stay on course. Sensei provide tactical direction to long-term visioning, produce faster results because of their experience, and set higher expectations allowing for higher achievement.

An organization can hire an external sensei or develop one from within; that decision depends on the needs of each organization and its culture and practices. In either case the sensei will need the backing of the rest of the management team. The sensei should be focused solely on lean and report directly to the highest levels of the organization to ensure that leaders are prepared to teach and lead by lean principles and practices and to send the message that the improvement effort is important. If the sensei is external to the organization, then the cost can be substantial. Although improvement activities can generate significant return on investment (see Chapter 4), it makes sense to leverage sensei time heavily at first for teaching but, over time, to develop this expertise in-house and to free the sensei for coaching and more complex lean applications. It can also be helpful to have outside eyes measuring progress. Sensei can help an organization gain early momentum and maintain the discipline needed to set stretch targets and compel the work needed for attainment of goals. HHC chose an external consulting group with deep roots in lean, many choose similar firms, and others choose independent, experienced teachers or sensei who came to them with decades of experience in manufacturing, aerospace, or other service industries.

Lean thinking is truly a new way of doing business. Of course, some *could* do this without an internal/external sensei, but those are the exceptional few. The literature shows us that the majority of groups fail within 2 years of attempting a lean transformation, often in part because of the failure to invest resources and time into building a lean infrastructure, both human and process. Critical to future improvement is succession planning that includes leaders that have been trained by sensei in lean thinking to build a culture of learning.[10,11]

Lean in Health Care

In the most recent decade, lean has been rapidly moving into the health care industry and the public sector, including the United States Army and Veteran's Administration. It can be hard to see the adaptation of lean in health care; how care flows through a health care organization is typically fragmented (between providers, buildings, and institutions). A lean practitioner needs to learn to "see waste," create continuous flow and transition from batch, and queue to one-by-one flow. Seeing waste is a learned skill. However, when comparing a product family approach for establishing end-to-end flow in manufacturing to clinical pathway families in health care, there are a lot of similarities regarding how this strategy can drastically improve the various flows in health care. Look at the entire end-to-end flow of how psychiatric care is provided for a patient from being seen in the psychiatric emergency room, admission to an inpatient bed, through discharge, and ultimately to aftercare in outpatient services. The traditional flow is typically viewed as unconnected silos or departments, without tight connections to pull the patient along their care continuum.

In the health care world, we have much experience with various improvement strategies and tools and are wary of the "new initiative." Only recency of arrival to the field foretells how many and which of these tools we have tried, tested, and often put aside. In fact, many of these tools, including Quality Circles, Total Quality Management, Failure Mode Effects Analysis, and the ubiquitous Plan-Do-Study-Act (PDSA), are integral to TPS. So why lean? Lean borrows from all of the tools we have used singularly and often sequentially in the past and vests them in a compelling system of improvement. It offers a means to create value and eliminate waste that is accessible to everyone in an organization, and, unlike most traditional improvement efforts, is not solely the purview of quality departments or committees, physicians, and nurses. Improvement activities are not conducted by a small group of experts; rather, all employees are encouraged to participate in daily and periodic activities toward the resolution of locally defined problems. Tools and tactics range from the simple to the complex and are generally learned by a rolling cadre of individuals who gradually become reabsorbed by the organization and serve to continue to embed lean knowledge and practices. Many organizations spread the improvements more deeply throughout the institution, gradually changing the organizational culture to better focus on patient needs and systematize underlying principles. The latter is often considered a "lean transformation" and requires long-term commitment from visionary leaders.

In health care, waste is rampant. Anyone who has waited for an appointment in a crowded doctor's office, filled out three forms that ask for the same information, or worse, been the recipient of a medication error, has experienced this. In manufacturing, lean has been in active use for more than 40 years. In *Lean Thinking*, Womack and Jones describe results from a number of companies, including Wiremold, a maker of wire management systems (75% reduction in time to market for new products, 20% annual increase in productivity), and Pratt and Whitney, maker of aircraft engines (growing from a loss of $283 million in 1992 to profits of more than $500 million in 3 years). Jeff Liker notes in *The Toyota Way* that Toyota produces cars in 12 months or less, as opposed to the typical 2- to 3-year process of other auto manufacturers. Closer to home, we learned that Dr. Patricia S. Gabow, former CEO of a sister public hospital system, Denver Health, had begun to realize savings and new revenue of over $10 million in less than 2 years of lean activity.[12]

It is often said that the definition of insanity is doing the same thing and expecting different results. In health-care, we needed radical change, and for that, pulling from outside of our industry for solutions was an unconventional strategy that seemed as extreme as our situation. Our developing improvement system includes a nascent daily management system, an approach to the achievement of business goals, a vehicle for staff engagement, and an extensive set of accessible tools that unite to ensure that value, as defined by the customer (in our case, the patient), is provided when and where needed, in the right quantity, efficiently and reliably. Lean itself is founded on two essential and undeniable principles: respect for people and society and continuous improvement for the patient, the supplier, and the staff member. Supportive planning tools, such as *hoshin kanri* or strategy deployment, enable strategic alignment within departments and between departments, within hospitals, and between the myriad entities that comprise today's health care systems. A process improvement structure such as this is a natural fit in the health care industry and, we have found, is particularly well suited for behavioral health. Its process orientation, rigorous application of scientific method, and focus on enabling people touches the part of us that brought many of us to a helping profession in the first place. Organizations that consistently apply a structured system of process improvement over time are willing to set ambitious goals, unleash creativity, and practice a disciplined approach to continuous learning achieve high levels of performance.[13,14]

When HHC initiated lean we met with our union partners to discuss our plans and gain their insights regarding staff concerns and considerations. To this audience of 13 local union representatives and leaders, the concept of applying an improvement system developed by a non-union car manufacturer to a public hospital system was not an intuitive match. Although its effectiveness in manufacturing wasn't questioned, many of the representatives questioned the relevance of a car-making system to a patient care organization. "Patients aren't cars." We provided the limited outcome data we had available to us and talked about how other hospitals had begun to use this approach to accumulate significant benefits in clinical care, operations, and the financial bottom line. Still wary, our union's sin qua non is patient care. Their initial, guarded support was couched in a small wisdom: "Don't call this thing lean. It sounds like a layoff plan." Shortly thereafter, lean at HHC became *Breakthrough, the HHC Enterprisewide Improvement System*. Today, *Breakthrough* is the term of art in our organization. Throughout this book, however, we use the word "lean" for purposes of clarity and generalizability for the reader.

The Etiology of Lean at New York City Health and Hospitals Corporation

Various analyses have estimated that the number of health care organizations that have adopted lean in the United States runs at less than 4%. Virginia Mason Medical Center in Seattle, Washington, is the first well-documented hospital system in the United States to adopt lean. Gary Kaplan, chief executive officer of Virginia Mason, describes two consecutive years of unprecedented financial losses and significant concerns about quality of care as the events that drove his organization to make radical, system-wide, and deep improvements beginning in 2001.[15] Health care institutions come to lean for many reasons and in many forms, sometimes tragic, sometimes economic, sometimes led by an insurgent group of innovators, or sometimes a search for the next competitive edge.

A case could be made for different improvement systems. HHC's extensive clinical quality improvement program has relied on the Deming cycle of Plan-Do-Study-Act for years, but we never perceived of this well-worn tool as more than a method for working through specific quality issues. We briefly looked at Six Sigma but passed it up as requiring a level of specialization that would limit participation. Certainly, our own experience using simple PDSA cycles, Total Quality Management, and some of the strategies mentioned later in this chapter bore great successes for HHC. Perhaps the essential ingredients—a platform upon which to practice effective and varied tools so that a culture of expectation (for big results, for testing and experimenting), of continuous learning, of humility that allows us to learn from others, and of an appreciation for iterative improvement—could be mastered through other means for some organizations. For HHC, it took lean to motivate us to dig deeper than tools and spot improvement and to change the way we lead, manage, and "do."

Living this view is difficult, thus most of us come to it only because our "platforms" truly are afire and we stick with it only because we believe the promise of, and begin to reap, tremendous benefits in quality, safety, patient satisfaction, staff performance and engagement, cost reduction and revenue enhancement, and productivity and effectiveness the likes of which we have not before experienced.

HHC's struggles to move past a series of disconnected and all-too-often short-term successes could be traced to the early to mid-1990s, when several of our hospitals lost or were threatened with the loss of accreditation and a new mayoral administration questioned the need for the city's aged public hospital system. After years of dependence on the City of New York for financial assistance and facing claims of poor-quality care, HHC was struggling to maintain morale and fight the image of a mismanaged, bloated bureaucracy providing care of questionable quality when, with a new mayor, the city sought to sell or bring in a private management company to operate parts of the system. HHC and its member hospitals have always had their critics as well as their supporters and, at that time, HHC was not the only public hospital system struggling for survival. Although Medicaid had traditionally been considered a poor payer, reductions in private insurance reimbursements and rising fixed costs suddenly meant that the public hospitals were competing for patients the private sector had largely ignored in the past. Public hospitals were closing all over the country. Even then, HHC was the largest municipal hospital system in the country, and the role of the public sector in providing direct health care was being questioned by policy makers and taxpayers in many locales.

The city's position was a rallying cry for many people within and outside of HHC, and the mayor, even while actively working to at least reduce the size of the system, entrusted care of HHC to a physician whose long history as an HHC employee and corporate level manager gave him internal credibility and a mandate to restructure the corporation's financial relationship with the city toward financial independence. While the city argued its case to sell or contract out the management of individual hospitals to a private entity in court, Dr. Luis Rojas Marcos led a major financial reorganization effort, analyzing the cost and revenue side of the business, reducing the size of the budget, and making the hard decision to lay off staff. Importantly, for the first time, Dr. Marcos insisted that we could increase patient revenue without violating HHC's treasured mission. For many HHC employees, asking the patient for financial or insurance information was blasphemous. Staff is deeply devoted to patients, many of whom have significant health concerns and complicated lives. Requiring patients to submit co-pays and be fee-scaled seemed picayune and unfair, especially within the context of HHC's historic relationship with the city, through which supplementary funds were expected each year. It took several years for staff, long equating our proud mission, "to serve all regardless of ability to pay" with "free" care, to begin to feel comfortable requiring that all patients participate in financial counseling to determine insurance eligibility. Over time, and supported by a generous and comprehensive self-pay policy, recognition that the historic mission was endangered by an unsustainable financial model led to routine application of basic revenue cycle requirements, and ultimately, HHC's finances were in the black for the first time in recorded history. In the process, we learned an important lesson that would drive us to greater accomplishments over the next 15 years: We could make change across the system to a heretofore unimaginable level by engaging employees across the system in the identification and resolution of problems.

HHC is a "quasi-mayoral agency" established by state statute in 1969 with a board of directors appointed by the mayor and inclusive of individuals designated by the city council and a chief executive appointed by this board. For most of its history, turnover in senior positions was frequent and destabilizing. With Dr. Marcos' relatively extended term (from 1995 through 2002), he became the longest tenured president in the organization's history, and senior leadership across the system had the opportunity to mature together. Upon his departure, another physician with deep roots in HHC was appointed president and a well-planned and comprehensive hand-off set up Dr. Benjamin K. Chu to continue a focus on system stabilization and improvement. Dr. Chu, although remaining in his position for only 3 years, used his extensive contacts throughout the system and his credibility as a primary care internist, attending physician, and chief medical officer at the hospital and corporate level to rally the organization to build on the financial stability Dr. Marcos had achieved.

Working with the Institute for Healthcare Improvement (IHI), Dr. Chu brought the concept of team-based learning to HHC. Serving a largely low-income, ethnic minority population and located in neighborhoods with the highest rates of ambulatory care–sensitive conditions in the city, HHC serves a disproportionate volume of patients with uncontrolled diabetes, asthma, and heart conditions. Using the IHI model of "learning collaboratives," multidisciplinary teams of physicians, nurses, nutritionists, social workers, and administrators from each hospital and health center began to meet regularly to share best practices for the treatment of chronic conditions, to measure improvements in health outcomes, and to develop standards for the elimination of hospital-acquired infections.

These collaboratives, led by Dr. Karen Scott Collins, had phenomenal results, and the level of achievement often outperformed state and national averages. By 2008, more than 50,000 patients were being tracked in the HHC Diabetes Registry, enabling care coordination and targeted care that resulted in 45.5% of adult diabetic patients having blood sugar levels, blood pressure, and cholesterol in healthy ranges. The number of children enrolled in MetroPlus (HHC's health maintenance organization) who had emergency room visits resulting from asthma fell by 6% and related hospital admissions fell by 25% over a 5-year period ending in 2011. The American Diabetes Association estimates that the 2012 cost of diabetes in the United States was $245 billion, 41% more than the previous study in 2007. On average, a diagnosis of diabetes was associated with medical costs that were two to three times higher than the cost of care for individuals without diabetes.[16]

The rates of ventilator-associated pneumonia (VAP) in our intensive care units (ICUs) dropped to 1.2 in 2011 from 10.5 in 2005, indicating that this success was sustained. Of 27 adult ICUs, 22 went 5 months or more without a VAP, with 11 of the 27 having no VAP cases for the whole of 2011. The incidence of VAP is also associated with longer hospital stays, including longer stays in ICUs. The cost of caring for a patient who acquires a VAP has been identified as more than three times the cost (between $11,000 and $57,000 per patient episode) of a critical care patient who does not acquire pneumonia.

These results were evidence that, indeed, we could improve the quality of patient care while lowering the total cost of care. We also learned something else that fueled our growing confidence—interdisciplinary teamwork and bringing teams together to share ideas breeds a healthy competition that begets higher performance.

While the collaboratives continued, two additional efforts helped to further redefine HHC. Under the direction of Marlene Zurack, the corporate chief financial officer, a process of financial microanalysis began to move across the system. Site by site, teams of staff within local finance offices selected specific revenue cycle and budgeting problems and worked together to solve these. Simultaneously, a corporate-wide effort, labeled the ambulatory care restructuring initiative, sought to reduce cycle times, waits for appointments, and no-show rates. Over 6 years, across 127 primary care clinics throughout the system, the average wait for appointments, appointment cycle times, and no-show rates dropped substantially, as indicated in Figure 1.1.[17]

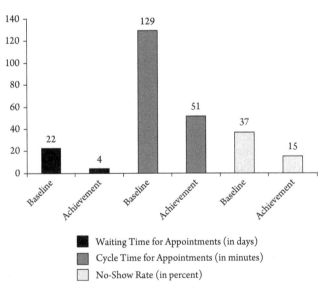

Waiting Time for Appointments (in days)
Cycle Time for Appointments (in minutes)
No-Show Rate (in percent)

Note: Baseline data is from 2002; Achievement data is from 2008

Figure 1.1 Enterprisewide Ambulatory Care Restructuring Initiative. Source: NYCHHC Office of Corporate Planning and HIV Services.

These efforts and the burgeoning patient safety work led by Caroline Jacobs repeatedly demonstrated the power of working in teams across and within sites, of shared learning, and bottom-up problem solving.

However, many of these efforts ultimately succumbed to the same villain. Years of work could be too quickly undone. The constant emergence of new priorities, some of our own making, and many imposed by the increasingly competitive and volatile financial and regulatory environments in which we existed, were distracting and pulled resources away from our improvement work. We had learned the importance of data—to establish a floor from which to improve and to demonstrate the effectiveness of applied strategies—but the burden of data collection and measurement fell to the same individuals already tasked with operations and clinical care and was too often inadvertently sabotaged by competing demands for time. When key personnel changes took place, it became clear that sustaining improvements was too often dependent on specific people rather than the adoption of accepted standards. We needed a buttress against our own vulnerabilities and the external tumult that would bring us the technical ability to spread and sustain change.

Enter Lean

In 2006, at the IHI National Forum, the improvement conference held by IHI each December, HHC was introduced to lean. A group of individuals from HHC participated in a workshop conducted by our sister public hospital Denver Health, led by the indefatigable Patricia Gabow. Dr. Gabow recited the story of Denver Health's inspiring lean journey and the results they were achieving with lean. The HHC participants came back to New York urging that we bring this process to HHC. The corporate office responded by undertaking an evaluation and procurement process that resulted in the selection of the lean consulting firm, Simpler North America, L.P., and in November 2007, our journey began in earnest.

Health Care's Burning Platform

The first step we take to improve any aspect of our work is to agree on the definition of the problem. In lean lexicon, this problem statement is articulated in the first box of a summary, one-page document called an A3. [18] We call this statement our "burning platform." In health care, the ultimate burning platform is a threat to patient safety, the potential for patient harm, or even death. At HHC, at the corporate level our improvement work is motivated by our knowledge that we are capable of doing much better; that our patients deserve the best, safest care; and that our survival quite literally depends on an organizational transformation wherein all staff are part of a solution. The IHI collaboratives, process redesign, and Six Sigma are only some of the tools health care systems have applied to these concerns. With the publication of *To Err Is Human: Building a Safer Health System* (National Academy Press, November 1999) and the launch of the *100,000 Lives Campaign* initiated by the Institute for Healthcare Improvement in 2004, the frequency and indeed, in some cases, the probability that hospitalization poses the risk of harm or death from receiving the wrong dose of medication, poor communication between hospital personnel, or a failure to wash hands caught the attention of health care institutions and the public at large. Our self-image as "helpers" was sorely challenged by the report's finding that as many as 98,000 individuals are victims of medical errors each year.

Adding to this humbling realization, as participants in the larger health care system, we had come to expect as inevitable some level of harm (i.e., Does an airplane pilot "expect" she will bring down some percentage of the planes she flies?), health reform emerged as an essential conversation in the United States. The transition from payment based on the volume of services provided to regular payment of a flat monthly fee to cover all expenses incurred for treatment of a patient, regardless of cost, has forced health care providers to attempt to move the locus of care to outpatient and preventive services, eliminate unnecessary tests and invest in community health, or to develop niches that allow them to continue to be competitive for high-revenue, specialty services.

By late 2008, only a year after adopting lean as its enterprise-wide improvement system, HHC found itself with a deficit of $1.2 billion and embarked on a restructuring plan to make significant cost reductions through contracting the management of certain support services, allowing attrition to reduce the workforce and restructuring major services, such as perioperative services, housekeeping, and laundry. To affect these cost reduction strategies while maintaining a commitment to "no layoffs due to lean activity," clear lines of demarcation were drawn between any activities related to workforce reduction and lean activities.

Hospitals are not immune from the fad of the moment, and the goal of providing excellence in care is not new either. Awards for quality and innovation are numerous. Since the adoption of quality circles, total quality management, Plan-Do-Check-Act (PDCA), Plan-Do-Study-Act (PDSA), balanced scorecards, Team STEPPS, collaborative learning, and myriad other processes to improve clinical and operational quality, hospitals have been frustrated by the challenge of creating systemic improvement within large institutions with multiple stakeholders and competing interests. Although inarguably some quality tactics have produced positive results, many have a relatively short shelf life and practitioners struggle with spread and sustainment.[19] At HHC, despite the 6 years we invested in ambulatory care redesign and the strong results we achieved, we found that data integrity had diminished considerably at the 10-year point, and the results we'd achieved several years earlier in some cases were not sustained and were obscured in others.

Health care practitioners are not, by definition, any more ready for change than other professionals, and as of this writing, lean is practiced in only a small but growing minority of the health care institutions in the United States. These organizations are pioneers and risk takers whose missions and organizational cultures embrace the principles of respect for people and society and continuous improvement. In a meta-analysis of studies of quality management programs, Asif and de Bruijn identify failure modes of quality programs. The authors found that, frequently, traditional quality programs consist of tools alone; their application is not vested in a clear linkage to business strategy, and they were often isolated from the routines and structures that act as the repository of organizational knowledge that nurtures a common culture (rather than various subcultures). The intent of quality managers related to program implementation (i.e., performance improvement or legitimization in the eyes of stakeholders) also determines the success or failure of such efforts.[20]

Lean doesn't promise quick fixes or complex formulas but, rather, a lifelong journey of incremental improvement toward zero defects. Perhaps hospitals that gravitate toward iterative, long-term strategies, and certainly those that succeed, are those able to take a long view and are led by individuals who clearly articulate a vision and support the development of the organization's people. In *Good to Great*, Jim Collins notes that this "servant leadership" is a common trait that separates the good from the great leader.[21] This path requires behavior change at many levels and, in health care, can not only lead to improvements in care, operations, and financial health but can address significant regulatory and competitor pressures to demonstrate high levels of patient and staff satisfaction. Lean holds the added attraction of providing a large number of powerful yet simple tools that are well received and employable by a wide variety of staff.

Across the country, hospital operating margins tend to be lower than other industries, with an average of less than 4%. In New York City, where operating margins hover at less than 0%, 15 hospitals have closed since 2000.[22,23] Hospitals that can survive the continuing financial pressures of the recession of the last several years, coupled with the complete restructuring of the payment and service systems, will have to re-make themselves in ways we are only beginning to understand. To some of us, lean provides a new way of doing business.

Making the Case

Learning how to effectively apply the tools and principles of lean is only a part of the equation when transforming any organization or even a set of processes. Establishing a culture in which all employees, including front-line workers, managers, and leaders, are engaged in transparent problem-solving is the other half of the equation. The first step toward establishing this environment is to articulate and continuously communicate the burning platform that describes why the lean transformation work is required, and how each person within the organization can have a favorable impact on the change needed. If the compelling reason for change is not established, then the people in the organization will not feel a sense of urgency. Change is much easier and more likely to succeed if people understand and buy into why it is so important. Another key element of establishing a lean culture is the requirement of the executive leadership team to lead by example, by participating in lean events such as value stream analysis events and rapid improvement events. It is much easier to set expectations of engaged participation for the organization when people see their key leaders submitting themselves to the lean process. This hands-on approach is known as the "dirty hands university," which is another way of saying you have to learn by doing. Further, leadership teams at every level of the organization must actively engage in walking the gemba, the "place where the work is done," on a regular basis to discover which elements of the lean transformation are working well and which are not working so well. This direct interaction with staff and the observation of processes in the workplace are the only ways to really understand the truth, whether good, bad, or even ugly.

Lean has only been applied to health care for about 10 years. Some of the early lean adopters had no choice but to learn from other industries, such as manufacturing and hospitality, because there simply were no models in the sector. Virginia Mason went to Japan and studied air conditioners being built. Thedacare watched lawnmowers and snow blowers being built, and Denver Health brought on an advisory board with representatives from FedEx and Marriott. Today, with lean applications in health care approaching 10 years, those of us who want to learn from our peers can turn to a growing number of lean hospitals but most often still turn to these three pioneers to see more mature applications and "what good looks like." Lean development is slow and iterative; the sharing of insights characteristic of lean organizations is comforting and inspiring to those of us who are earlier on our journey. It helps that organizations that were already innovating were some of the first to adopt lean and were already playing the role of "best practice" in the sector. Look at the Cleveland Clinic (cardiac care), Park Nicollet (zero based budgeting), Johns Hopkins (research), and Kaiser Permanente (Web-based access to patient records). Perhaps 5% of hospitals in the United States have begun to use lean tools. Lean is hard to do, and it gets harder until it becomes thoroughly embedded in an organization whose workforce and systems are transformed. Those hospitals that stick with it over time are going to be those that exhibit the rare blend of strong and dedicated leadership, an awakened, team-based workforce, a burning platform and healthy doses of persistence, good luck, and timing.

Building Breakthrough, the New York City Health and Hospitals Enterprise-wide Improvement System

In 2007, when our lean journey began, we could not imagine the daily work we would take on—how what we did each day would change, what it would look like.

But we did have a vision of a "transformed" system, a public hospital system in which everyone was a "problem solver," in which every employee was valued and contributed value to the system each day and in which value, as defined by the patient, was what we delivered.

We brought in consultants who promised an approach closely aligned with the Toyota Production System to teach us a system of principles, values and tools for improvement, elimination of waste, and engagement of people. (These are covered in more detail later in this chapter.) Originally, we aimed at a rollout across at least all of the largest hospitals, health centers, long-term care facilities, and subsidiaries (23) we operated within 3 years. In the first year, we worked with six sites, and by the end of the third year we had reached only an additional seven. As eager as we were for all of these larger entities to adopt lean quickly, we learned we needed to "slow down to go faster."

The first several sites were pulling hard to get going—they had big issues they wanted to address and were convinced that lean would help them do this. Our commitment to responding only to pull (rather than "push" lean on sites), and not requiring sites to join in by a certain date, lead some to rush forward, whereas others took a wait-and-see position. Sites that came forward first were phenomenal in their uptake of lean methods and vision for the future. Those that were reluctant had reasons to hesitate. In an organization (and sector) that had a long history of chasing sequential next best things, was lean just the newest fiction cooked up by the corporate office, or a fad that would fade with the upcoming citywide election or crisis de jour? Eventually, by year 4, more sites came knocking as word got out about the results early adopters achieved and these successes were celebrated. By the end of year 4, 14 sites were live and 5 more were eager to start. We have learned a lot from what is now 19 start-ups and work to incorporate these learnings with each new start. Although with each new insight we learn how little we know and how much farther we have to travel, elements of what is becoming a system are gradually becoming more routine and more widely adopted throughout the organization.

Our typical start-up and cycle of activity looks like that described in Figure 1.2. We now precede the launch of a site with a series of planning discussions and ask leadership to complete basic lean training, ensure that at least a "Breakthrough deployment officer" and two facilitators are on board, and provide training regarding roles and responsibilities and basic tools to a core group of leaders and senior managers. Support is provided to the facility before the kick-off in the form of a dedicated teacher, or sensei, for up to several months to begin to develop visual management boards for site-wide and area specific management and to provide 1:1 training and support to the leadership and Breakthrough team. This "pre-launch" period also provides an opportunity for the sensei to learn about the facility so that early guidance is provided in context. Executives are encouraged to participate in events taking place at other HHC sites and, with a list of

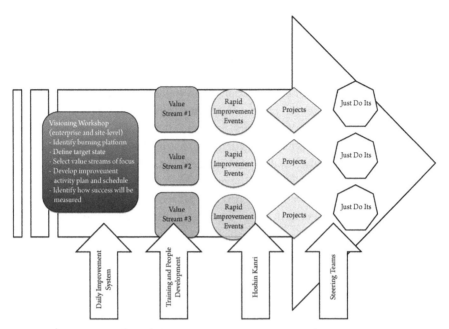

Figure 1.2 Elements of Breakthrough, the HHC Enterprisewide Improvement System.
Source: Enterprise Steering Committee Monthly Report, December 2012.

recommended lean books, form reading groups. Key point sheets that identify these steps are shared with sites and used to bring the site to the launch date ready for a strong start-up and able to maximize the learning opportunities of the first several months.

The formal launch of lean at each site starts with a half-day executive Breakthrough workshop, attended by site executives and union leadership. An overview of the corporation's lean journey, plans and results, as well as the approach, tools, and tactics that together define a large part of the visible, technical aspects of lean is provided. The following 2 days are spent in a visioning workshop to define improvement goals and areas for initial focus. This session is attended by a smaller group of site leaders, including administrators and physicians. Within a month, value stream mapping takes place in the areas selected, and a monthly cadence of week-long rapid improvement events follows.

To ensure that lean work is conducted in areas of value to the local facilities, HHC sites are encouraged to select two "value streams" for initial improvement work that are of the greatest urgency locally. A value stream is all of the activities, both value-added and non-value-added, required within an organization to deliver a specific service—"everything that goes into" creating and delivering the "value" to the end customer, typically defined as a patient. HHC's larger sites, including most hospitals, frequently select emergency departments, perioperative services, inpatient flow, ambulatory care, or mental health services when they first start out. Because any value stream is rife with waste (Liker claims that most business processes are 90% waste; Koenigsaeker goes even farther, stating the norm is as high as 95%), lean practitioners work through value stream processes through multiple passes. It takes time to reduce layers of waste, from the obvious (like waiting room queues) to the more subtle (such as accepting mediocre results). As layers are peeled away, more waste, and more stubbornly adherent waste, is gradually revealed. It also takes time to understand which value streams truly provide the greatest opportunity for improvement versus simply affect the most pain. And although specific value streams may be descoped from an overly broad initial definition over time, most HHC facilities end up working through these first value streams for at least several years with occasional and sometimes extended breaks for changes in leadership or external distractions.

When HHC initiated its lean effort, the first priority was to create improvement momentum and ownership and to develop a means for engaging the workforce in transformative activity. Over time, the need and desire to learn from each other and avoid remaking the wheel has grown and the organization's burning platform became about survival when an unprecedented deficit grew out of a combination of government payment reform, significant increases in pension costs and increases in care to the uninsured during the economic downturn. At that point, about 2 years in, leaders from across HHC asked that each site focus on one of two high-impact services—perioperative and emergency services—and/or at least one revenue-generating area.

Comprehensive mapping of the current state allows us to identify all of the specific activities occurring along the value stream or service line, represented pictorially and flowing from left to right. We map to see waste, unevenness, and overburden in existing processes; then create a target state map to size the opportunity; share a vision and communicate it visually; create a future in which wastes are removed so that value can flow uninterrupted from end to end; and acknowledge permission to change and commit to results. In a value stream analysis (VSA), a team of people who work in the process to be mapped join with suppliers to the process and people new to the process ("fresh eyes") to identify the specific steps that comprise the value stream. The resulting "map" allows discovery of waste in all manner of processes and functions. As we become better cartographers, the maps become more data-driven and, as such, more useful and are typically represented as large, wall-sized visual tools. During the VSA, we identify specific problems to be solved through Rapid Improvement Events (RIEs; a.k.a. kaizen events), projects, or "just do its." Our RIE is a 4.5-day process utilizing a team-based methodology and applying lean tools for seeing waste, testing solutions, and making improvements during the course of the event. The RIEs are scoped during the VSA and are scheduled over a 6- to 12-month period. RIEs have been the primary

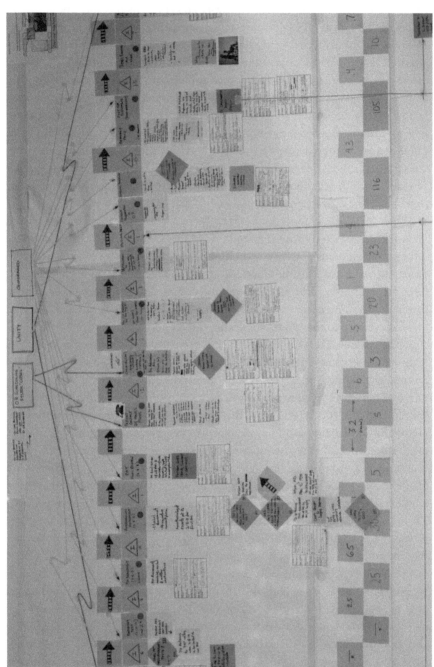

Figure 1.3 Value stream map.

process change mechanism we have used to date. An example of a value stream map is included as Figure 1.3.

During the first year, HHC hospitals were expected to produce two RIEs a month for the first 6 months and move gradually to between four and six events a month. By the end of 2 years, a comfortable cadence of up to eight events a month was initially expected. At the smaller health centers, a limit of one or two events a month was reasonable, given the small size of staff in any one value stream and the impact of taking a team of staff off line for a week at a time for events. Some sites met and exceeded this pace, whereas others settled at a much lower rate of production because of unique, competing priorities, more skeptical leadership, or professional biases.

Our focus on RIEs was purposeful. Spending 4.5 days with a team of opinionated people who are empowered to fix problems that may have existed for years is a set-up for conflict. Even for the seasoned team member, it is a struggle to use "creativity over capital" to solve long-standing problems, to loosen the stranglehold of "we've always done it that way" from individuals who are not sure that giving something up—even if it is widely seen as ineffective—won't result in more work. Through this process, however, team members have to work together for an extended period of time; enough time to express and work through what shorter processes leave unresolved. By mid-week, the team creates and tests solutions to the problems they have defined. Through this cycle of testing the team can review the results of their work, modify their solutions as needed, and put the tested and successful solutions in place before the end of the week. "Rapid improvement," not "rapid planning," is the focus. The last day of the week is for celebration. We gather teams, learn what they have accomplished, and applaud our colleagues' good work. The experience of an RIE is one of the most powerful engagement tools lean offers. The length of the event and the specific processes the team members go through combine for a formula that encourages participants to pull from their reservoirs of patience and creativity, reduces inhibitions against communicating directly, and rewards them with fixes to long-standing problems. Examples of the process and results of specific rapid improvement events are provided in Chapters 5 through 9.

RIEs are conducted within a larger context of continuous improvement. HHC uses A3s, the metric nomenclature for a paper size equal to 11 x 17", to document plans, improvements, and problem-solving processes. "A3 thinking" is an organized, sequenced process that asks the user to define the reason for action, current and target states, gap analysis, solution approach, rapid experiments, completion plan, confirmed state, and insights or lessons learned. A3 thinking encourages consensus building, unifies culture around a simple systematic methodology, becomes a communication tool that follows a logical narrative, and builds over years as organizational learning matures.

Figure 1.4 provides an example of an A3, with numbers indicating the sequence of development, from Boxes 1 through 9. In this case, an A3 was used to articulate the "Transformation Plan of Care" (TPOC) for Kings County Hospital Center.

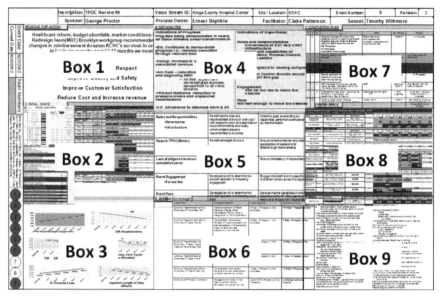

Figure 1.4 A3 Example. Box 1: Reason for action; Box 2: Initial state map; Box 3: Target state metrics; Box 4: Gap analysis and root cause; Box 5: Solutions; Box 6: Rapid experiments; Box 7: Completion plan; Box 8: Evidence of success; Box 9: Learning and insights. *NYCHHC 2012.*

The overall goal of many RIEs is to remove waste, create "flow," and develop "standard work." The flow we seek is the progressive achievement of tasks and/ or information as they proceed along the value stream without stops or rework. A focus on flow challenges the enterprise to reorganize the value stream to be continuous, without interruption from the patient's perspective. A streamlined nonstop experience for the patient is the goal.

Our standard work events range from identifying, documenting, and training staff to perform repeatable tasks without error, to complex analyses of workload, relative burden, and an agreed-upon set of work procedures that effectively combines people, materials, and machines to maintain quality, efficiency, safety, and predictability. The work itself is described precisely in terms of cycle time, work in process, sequence, task time, loading, layout, and the inventory needed to conduct the activity.

Ultimately, the type of event or activity—the tool—we use depends on the problem to be solved. Additional tools we have found helpful include the following:

Vertical value stream mapping, or VVSM, is a tool for scoping and driving major projects utilizing lean principles. VVSM enables "one-off" activities to flow without waste; it is used for improving "nonrecurring" processes; it works for highly complex processes and is a key enabler for multidisciplinary teams.

"2P," or process preparation, is used to redesign or design physical settings and programs. These events tend to be very hands-on and fun and can result in significant capital and resource savings.

In addition, we conduct many smaller events in a workshop setting, applying consistent A3 thinking and basic problem solving tactics to resolve less complex challenges in the moment.

By early 2012, the power of events was such that despite some unevenness, the pull by staff to participate in lean continued to grow across the corporation. Events were seen as innovative opportunities to make change in long-standing problems, to obtain attention and resources, to learn more about lean, and to gain recognition. It helped that, by this time, annual manager evaluations required demonstration of basic lean competencies and leaders were expected to participate in at least one event per year.

Oversight of lean effort is conducted primarily at the site level, through steering teams chaired by the site leader. An enterprise steering committee provides strategic guidance and general monitoring of corporate-wide progress. The A3s created by each site during their original visioning workshop are reviewed and amended as needed every 4 months with guidance from our external sensei. In the first few years, these site A3s included contributions toward enterprise-level financial and process measures. By the end of the third year, these system-level measures, and the process to monitor them, were reduced to financial outcomes and process counts as the concurrent measurement system for a major restructuring effort grew in significance, and the enterprise steering committee began to question the effectiveness and need for the role they played in oversight. At the end of 2012, the committee revised its charter and was reconstituted to address a growing desire to see a wider spread of improvements across sites, to ensure that lean work was strategically aligned with newly developed business goals and to support the further development of site improvement infrastructure with the express intent of reducing dependence on our external consultants.

Notes

1. Womack, JP, Jones DT. 1996. *Lean Thinking: Banish Waste and Create Wealth in Your Corporation*. New York: Simon & Schuster.
2. Liker, JK. 2004. *The Toyota Way*. New York: McGraw-Hill.
3. Koenigsaecker, G. 2009. *Leading the Lean Enterprise Transformation*. New York: Productivity Press, Taylor and Francis Group.
4. Census of U.S. Manufacturers—Lean Green and Low Cost. *Industry Week*, September 18, 2007. Online version accessed May 1, 2013. http://www.industryweek.com/companies-amp-executives/census-us-manufacturers-lean-green-and-low-cost.
5. Spear, Steven J. 2009. *The High-Velocity Edge*. New York; McGraw-Hill.

6. Abrahamson, E. 2000. Change without pain. In *Harvard Business Review on Leading Through Change* (pp. 127–140). Boston: Harvard Business School Publishing Corporation.

7. Liker J, Rother, M. 2011. *Why Lean Fails.* Lean Enterprise Institute. http://www.lean.org/common/display/?o=1738. Accessed May 1, 2013.

8. Chakravorty, S. 2010. Where Process-Improvement Projects Go Wrong. *Wall Street Journal*, January 25.

9. *Gemba* is a Japanese word variously translated as where value is created or where the work is done. Walking the gemba provides the opportunity to "go see" the current state and visualize how and what work is being done. Toyota chairman Fujio Cho describes this as "Go See, Ask Why, Show Respect."

10. Reliable Plant. TPM is most difficult of all lean tools to implement, Rubrich, Larry. Accessed February 15 2013 from http://www.reliableplant.com/Read/26210/tpm-lean-implement.

11. Kim CS, Spahlinger DA, Kin JM, Billi JE, Lean health care: What can hospitals learn from a world-class automaker? *Journal of Hospital Medicine* 2006;1(3):191–199.

12. Personal conversation with Patricia A. Gabow, MD, former chief executive officer of Denver Health and Hospital Authority.

13. Grunden, Naida. *The Pittsburgh Way to Efficient Healthcare, Improving Patient Care Using Toyota Based Methods.* Boca Raton, FL: CRC Press, 2008.

14. *Going Lean in Health Care.* 2005. IHI Innovation Series white paper, Institute for Healthcare Improvement, MA.

15. Institute for Healthcare Improvement, Annual National Forum on Quality Improvement in Health Care, 2007, Orlando, FL. Plenary. Gary S. Kaplan, MD, FACMPE, FACPE, chairman and CEO of the Virginia Mason Health System.

16. American Diabetes Association. Economic costs of diabetes in the U.S. in 2012. *Diabetes Care*, online version available March 6, 2013, http://care.diabetesjournals.org/content/early/2013/03/05/dc12-2625.full.pdf+html, accessed July 24, 2013.

17. HHC partnered with the New York–based Primary Care Development Corporation and their contractors, Coleman Associates and Murray Tantau and Associates on this multiyear project.

18. Named for the size (11 x 17") of the paper it is written on, an A3 is a foundational lean tool that documents the essential information needed to scope a problem, define the current context and the desired future state, analyze the gap between these two, identify and test solutions, and specify how success will be defined.

19. *Quality and Safety in Health Care* 2002;11:345–351 doi:10.1136/qhc.11.4.345. Intensive care unit quality improvement: A "how-to" guide for the interdisciplinary team. *Critical Care Medicine* 2006; 34(1):211–218.

20. Asif, M, Joost de Bruijn, E, Douglas, Alex, Fisscher, Olaf A.M. "Why quality management programs fail: A strategic and operations management perspective," *International Journal of Quality & Reliability Management* 2009; 26(8): 778–794.

21. Collins, JC. *Good to Great, Why Some Companies Make the Leap . . . and Others Don't.* New York, 2001.

22. The Deteriorating Financial Condition of New York City's Nonprofit Hospitals, and Its Effect on Capital Investment. A Hospital Watch Special Report, United Hospital Fund, 2008.

23. *Hospital Watch.* United Hospital Fund, February 2011.

2

Behavioral Health Care and Lean

JOANNA OMI, JOSEPH P. MERLINO, JOYCE B. WALE,

KRISTEN BAUMANN, OLGA DESHCHENKO, AND ANTONIO D. MARTIN

Behavioral health care differs dramatically from the practices and environment of medical care settings, from the role of the physician to the nature of hospitalizations in which patients tend to be ambulatory. As is evident in inpatient and emergency room settings, behavioral health care has largely been oriented toward interdisciplinary treatment teams. In outpatient programs, formal teams or some form of "split treatment" may be used. In either case the psychiatrist may perform the initial overall assessment, make a diagnosis, and prescribe and monitor medication. Another practitioner then may provide psychotherapy or ongoing care of the patient (or "recipient of care," "consumer," or any of the various other terms that signal the shift from a medical model to one that is consumer driven or patient centered). Although today's behavioral health physician assumes a largely paternalistic approach—determining what the problem is, what the solution is, and how to achieve the solution, including whose role it will be to play which part in the overall treatment plan—the extent and effectiveness of communication and coordination between patient and provider is variable and a movement is under way to change this to support a milieu that is patient centered and focused on wellness and recovery.

Increasingly, on an inpatient service, an interdisciplinary group comes together often, but not always, under the leadership of the physician to review his or her assessment of the issue at hand with the patient as well as goals to pursue to achieve "wellness" as defined by the patient/consumer, not the physician. This represents a not-so-subtle shift in the care paradigm and requires changes in an organization's approach. Lean provides tools to help determine what and where the gaps are in an organization's current way of doing business (the current state) contrasted with where it wants to be, or more often needs to be (the target state), in the increasingly competitive market for patients.

Lean is also helpful in reducing the waste that comes with role confusion and duplication of efforts not uncommon in behavioral health care settings (see Box 2.1). The team approach to care has many positives to commend, but at times it can be a struggle to maintain clearly distinct roles. Some roles are unique to a given discipline—for example, a nursing care plan is done by a nurse, coordination of aftercare by a social worker, or medical consultation with neurology by the physician. But there are also overlapping roles: Who is the primary therapist; who leads the community meeting; who speaks with the family; who leads in crisis intervention?

Box 2.1 **Respect for People: Creating an Efficient Workplace**

Rapid improvement events (RIEs) have been conducted to enable staff to work at the full function of their licensure, to eliminate non-value-added and redundant activities so that staff can spend more time with patients.

- At Kings County Hospital Center in Central Brooklyn, obtaining and entering information into the patient's electronic medical record upon admission was being done by multiple staff—psychiatrist, social worker, internist, and nursing staff. By modifying work sequences and roles for documentation of evaluation and assessments during the first 72 hours of the patient's stay, the average time per admission was reduced from 8.5 hours to 5.4 hours. This enabled providers to spend more time in face-to-face evaluations and patient care.
- An RIE team at Metropolitan Hospital Center in East Harlem sought to reduce the amount of time needed for medical coding staff to review the completeness of medical record documentation and coding of care. The team discovered that coding staff spent hours each week walking between care units and multiple medical record locations in the pursuit of needed information. By relocating and consolidating storage and filing areas, as well as setting up the coders' workspace in a U-shaped flow cell, a mile of travel was eliminated from the distance coders collectively had to travel each day.
- Patients at North Central Bronx Hospital had to wait too long for routine mammograms and, for those women who also needed breast sonograms, another extended wait was required between the two procedures. By analyzing staff roles and work processes, creating standard work to support integration with other services, and moving clerical staff to the breast imaging area to work directly with the ultrasound and mammogram technician team leaders, an RIE team raised the percentage of patients who received routine screening mammograms from 70% to 90% and reduced the wait between mammograms and sonograms by 83%.

Lean provides a process for clarifying roles and preparing the necessary standard work for the team in which every team member's role is clearly and unambiguously spelled out, as are the key steps each player is responsible for delivering. This elimination of wasteful overlap cuts time from practitioners' overworked schedules, allowing them to focus on their unique roles, and clarifies for the patient who is partnering with him or her for the various agreed-upon goals. All in all, the flow of care is streamlined while increasing the likelihood of achieving the agreed-upon goals of the team and, most important, the person they work for: the patient.

Another unique aspect of behavioral health versus medicine has to do with the hospitalized patient, who is typically up and about, dressed in street clothes, and expected to be a contributing and participating member of the inpatient community. This requires a different approach as pertains to patient flow, staff flow, medication and meal distribution, and patient activity, including therapeutic groups. How such a unit is designed, where different functions are to take place, what the schedule should be—each of these assessments and processes benefit from lean analysis focused on reducing steps walked, reducing delivery wait times, enhancing safety, and reducing untoward events.

For outpatients, split treatment and coordination of care need to be monitored to ensure that the various providers are "on the same page" of an agreed-upon treatment plan and paying special attention to any changes, mental status, or risk level so that appropriate interventions are made in a timely and safe manner. Again, lean assists in the identification of any gaps in the flow as well as where standard work can be added to optimize efficiencies and desired outcomes. Additional matters pertaining to scheduling, billing, and other "back office" functions also benefit from this approach, clarifying actual versus expected work functions and burdens; understanding and creating appropriate "pull" and work cells; visual management through hourly, daily, and monthly data analysis; and team-based problem solving.

Challenges faced by behavioral health providers and consumers not typically shared by their contemporaries on the general care side of health care include stigma, community partnering, wellness and recovery efforts, and the important roles played by family and friends. To address these challenges, our lean events have included representatives from the community, advocacy agencies, friends, and family. This gives the event the reality base it needs to be most helpful to the agency or provider planning service delivery transformation.

Some improvements are limited in scope to a single practice or procedure, such as securing and returning patient property without loss upon request. Alternatively, a transformative, system-wide approach can be as broad as to look at the entire value stream, as in a hospital or large clinical setting, or even a network of facilities, as in an enterprise value stream. Chapters 5 through 9 illustrate how the use of lean methodology can assist in planning across the continuum of mental health services, demonstrating that regardless of the practice setting, lean can offer rewarding outcomes from a solo practice to an entire corporate enterprise. Lean tools are provided to assist leaders and practitioners with the development of their vision as well as the formulation of a plan of action for turning that vision into reality.

Behavioral Health at the New York City Health and Hospitals Corporation

Health and Hospitals Corporation (HHC) is a well-regarded provider of behavioral health services, an active innovator, and a leader in the national movement to transform care from a symptom-based medical model to a more skills-based, rehabilitation- and recovery-oriented system of care. HHC's strategic vision assumes that consumers of our services, regardless of immigration status, want to have a supportive place to live, meaningful work, and good interpersonal connections with others.

HHC is the largest provider of behavioral health services in New York City. Operating 42% of adult-licensed inpatient beds, 43% of the child/adolescent inpatient beds, and 18% of the detoxification beds in the city, HHC provides approximately 1 million outpatient mental health and substance abuse visits annually. HHC is the health and mental health safety net for low-income and uninsured individuals in the city of New York, and our hospitals are the preferred destination of police officers when they determine that a detainee needs psychiatric evaluation. The behavioral health service line at HHC is comprehensive, consisting of a full continuum of care from community outreach to emergency and outpatient treatment and inpatient care. All of HHC's 11 acute care hospitals support psychiatric inpatient units, totaling more than 1,200 mental health beds. Five hospitals offer inpatient detoxification services.

Six HHC facilities, including Kings County Hospital, operate licensed comprehensive psychiatric emergency programs (CPEPs). The CPEPs include mobile crisis teams and extended observation units (beds designated for stabilization of patients over a maximum period of 72 hours after admission). The acute hospitals and larger community health centers of HHC offer a broad array of ambulatory treatment services across the city including day programs, rehabilitation, case management, medication assistance and treatment, and ongoing counseling and therapy services.

Behavioral health providers within HHC have made significant advances through lean in a relatively short period. Long accustomed to process-oriented treatment and team-based interventions, behavioral health providers distinguish themselves among others in health care as being particularly amenable to lean applications. HHC has sought to stay abreast of emerging, evidence-based practices and was one of the first major behavioral health providers in the country to develop outpatient, court-ordered treatment programs, to adopt newer psychotropic medications, including buprenorphine and other injectable psychiatric medications, and to recognize the benefits of consumer support in improving health outcomes. Our existing focus on measurement in a highly regulated environment in which extensive documentation is required, and our comfort with continuous process improvement, makes lean adoption a natural next step for many providers.

Within the field of Behavioral Health in general, there has been slow but steady progress in measuring quality and performance improvement. System-wide metrics, developed over time by consensus of the HHC facility psychiatry directors, served to coalesce improvement efforts around a few key concerns. Even before the groundbreaking lean work conducted at Kings County Hospital, and as part of an overall strategy to ensure that patients played an active role in defining and receiving services, efforts across HHC to become more patient centered were under way. These efforts included the development of an award-winning training Tool Kit entitled "Work from the Heart...Improving Patient Centered Care," which highlighted the need to refocus our efforts on consumer-defined need. Efforts to reduce the use of seclusion and restraints became a focus close to a decade ago and were driven by safety and regulatory concerns as well as a desire to return dignity to the patient (the "respect for people" principle). HHC changed the definition of seclusion and restraint from a treatment intervention to a restrictive intervention and treatment failure by using crisis de-escalation techniques and ensuring that the workforce was highly trained and philosophically aligned. Over time, a shift in staff belief was accomplished and was demonstrated by the application of a symptom-based model for rehabilitation, recovery, and consumer empowerment. A second area of focus for HHC has brought about additional change. More than a decade ago we introduced peer counselors by empowering consumers who have reached a point in their own recovery to be able to help others to participate in their treatment planning, which led the way toward providing more patient-centered care. Encouraged by an emerging focus on consumer empowerment expressed by the New York State Office of Mental Health and incorporating the training resources of the New York Association of Psychiatric Rehabilitation Services (NYAPRS), these peer counselors trained much of the HHC workforce to embrace these models of recovery.

With the introduction of lean to HHC, behavioral health leaders sought opportunities to apply new tools to the service. About a year in, an enterprise-wide review process identified the need to prepare for major changes to reimbursement for detoxification services that held significant revenue implications for HHC. This would be our first corporate-wide application of lean in behavioral health. It is important to note that in New York State, behavioral health services are highly regulated by separate mental health and substance abuse authorities. The state substance abuse agency, the Office of Alcohol and Substance Abuse Services (OASAS), promulgated new regulations and payment policies for inpatient detoxification. At that time, we estimated that HHC could lose significant revenue if we did not modify our services to meet these new requirements. Two corporate-wide events were held in the first several months of 2009 to address this problem. For both events, teams of subject matter experts, clinicians, reimbursement and administrative staff, and "fresh eyes" came together for 4.5 days to develop a new service model that would both continue to serve patients' needs and enable appropriate revenue capture.

The first event team reviewed the current state and mapped what type of staff provided which service at what point during the patients' stay. An ideal and future state mapping process revealed changes that could be made to improve efficiencies and performance toward an enhanced patient experience. The team reduced administrative burden by 35% by eliminating previously required forms; this improvement enabled staff to meet regulatory compliance standards for patient processing times and created the opportunity for staff to complete all medical necessity, transfer, and continuity documentation. This first team developed processes for establishing and documenting level of care determination and implemented a multitiered approach to service delivery that included observation, medical supervision, and medical management. The team further updated policies and protocols in the HHC Detox Practice Guidelines, developed protocols for education/transfer of uncomplicated opioid-dependent individuals, instituted use of a withdrawal assessment tool, provided related staff training, and, with help from finance staff, provided follow-up, onsite audits and technical assistance to ensure proper level of care determinations. Full transition to these new processes and systems took 18 months and affected a broad array of detox services.

In the interim, a second event was held to develop a communication strategy to ensure sites were aware of the new changes in detox units for the HHC workforce and patients. Although a strategy was created by the team, we were less successful in spreading it than we had hoped. In hindsight, we could have been better informed by voice of the customer, and more mindful of the existing communication strategies at each site. This strategy included development of written materials and a series of meetings and "town hall" events to ensure that all affected individuals were informed of the changes. These two corporate-level events helped us recognize that even when team composition is intentionally inclusive of affected site representatives, events that are conducted to *create plans* for change away from the physical location in which the change will be made, as opposed to events to *create change* onsite where the change is needed, may not result in the level of local ownership requisite for effective implementation and sustainment.

Our lean work enabled us to achieve and sustain an appropriately balanced mix of treatment days, as indicated in Figure 2.1.

At monthly and quarterly meetings of all clinical and administrative psychiatry directors across the corporation, the subject of lean began to emerge more frequently. Five facilities initiated lean within behavioral health departments. Many of the facility leadership expressed interest in learning about each other's events and progress. As a way to increase communication and foster a learning environment at corporate-wide behavioral health programs, for the past few years sharing of lean

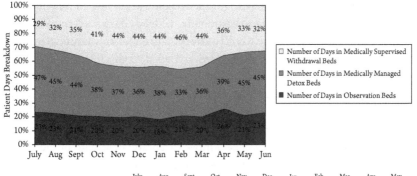

	July	Aug	Sept	Oct	Nov	Dec	Jan	Feb	Mar	Apr	May	Jun
Number Admitted/Transferred In	809	858	807	780	718	722	763	737	789	754	786	744

	July	Aug	Sept	Oct	Nov	Dec	Jan	Feb	Mar	Apr	May	Jun
Number of Days in Observation Beds	702	709	609	595	532	564	531	556	600	711	648	619
Number of Days in Medically-Managed Detox Beds	1,419	1,401	1,290	1,123	989	999	1,126	886	1,071	1,071	1,392	1,209
Number of Days in Medically-Supervised Withdrawal Beds	880	1,001	1,026	1,213	1,185	1,238	1,306	1,229	1,307	993	1,022	879

	July	Aug	Sept	Oct	Nov	Dec	Jan	Feb	Mar	Apr	May	Jun
Number of Days in Observation Beds	23.4%	22.8%	20.8%	20.3%	19.7%	20.1%	17.9%	20.8%	20.1%	25.6%	21.2%	22.9%
Number of Days in Medically-Managed Detox Beds	47.3%	45.0%	44.1%	38.3%	36.5%	35.7%	38.0%	33.2%	36.0%	38.6%	45.5%	44.7%
Number of Days in Medically-Supervised Withdrawal Beds	29.3%	32.2%	35.1%	41.4%	43.8%	44.2%	44.1%	46.0%	43.9%	35.8%	33.4%	32.5%

IN 2008, PRIOR TO DETOX REDESIGN, 100% OF PATIENTS WERE MEDICALLY MANAGED

Figure 2.1 Corporate Detox FY11 PAS Reported Patient Days—Growth and Stability Achieved in Medically Supervised Days. Source: NYCHHC Office of Behavioral Health Services.

practices has been regularly scheduled, usually around a theme associated with the program. For example, one corporate program focused on reducing length of stay and readmissions. Three facilities presented their Breakthrough work with a focus on outcomes and progress. One example of the benefit of integration of these reporting sessions has been greater understanding across sites of work being done to reduce the average length of stay for adult psychiatric patients in keeping with clinical need. With individual sites reporting strategies to understand and address delays in discharge, other sites are incited to conduct similar work and a plan to identify "least waste, best known way today" for corporate-wide adoption is under development. Future plans include creating an ongoing communication strategy to share events and outcomes among all facilities and encourage the broader use of lean.

Executive Leadership—The Facility View

Kings County Hospital Center introduced lean in its behavioral health services in 2008 in advance of bringing it to the greater facility out of the urgent need for radical change. At that time, the hospital had experienced the tragic death of a patient and a pre-existing investigation of behavioral health services by the federal Department of Justice was escalated as a result. Ms. Green, a patient of the hospital, died while waiting to be seen in the KCHC psychiatric emergency room. Security footage of the event provided alarming evidence that the facility could not simply deploy its existing improvement processes to ameliorate the circumstances that surrounded the tragedy. Indeed, deep and transformative attitude and behavioral change would be needed to effectively remodel processes and procedures for enduring change toward a safe and clinically appropriate environment.

The hospital executives who stepped in at this point had a difficult job on their hands. Not only were patient safety and management oversight under scrutiny, but KCHC Behavioral Health Services (BHS) was preparing at that time for a highly anticipated and symbolically significant move to a brand new, state-of-the-art facility while under the microscope of the Department of Justice, state and federal regulators, and patient advocacy groups. Demoralization among employees was widespread. Several new leaders were brought in and this team recognized that employees did not actively share ideas with each other, and many felt that their input was not valued. Although they worked side by side, people rarely grasped the challenges of each other's daily responsibilities. Lack of collaboration and direct communication between doctors, nurses, clerks, and administrators created an atmosphere in which going about business as usual was much easier than initiating improvement efforts.

Senior staff, some of whom were new to the facility, were relieved to find an approach to system transformation and process improvement in lean. They understood that staff generally felt unable to tackle what seemed to be overwhelming problems and the constant presence of regulators, advocates, and the Department of Justice was chilling. They believed intuitively that team-based problem solving would be effective in their environment, and resources—in the form of dedicated staff and an external sensei (in this case, an outside consultant expert in lean)— were made available to the hospital by the corporate office. Shortly after the adoption of lean, the new chief executive initiated a campus-wide customer service campaign designed after the Marriot program and mandated 100% participation. These two decisions—to enable staff to fix problems and to provide a constant backdrop of expectation regarding customer focus—had an immediate impact. A sense of being listened to and of being able to participate in decision making as well as a no-nonsense commitment to transparency and accountability created a sense of joint purpose, esprit de corps, and urgency to resolve long-standing problems. Over time, lean reached deeply enough throughout the institution that a palpable difference in attitude could be felt in the halls.

With lean rolling across the behavior health service, surveys began to show that staff recognized their positive contribution to the life of the hospital. The positive experience of rapid improvement events (RIEs) produced a sense of camaraderie that outlasted the duration of a lean event. Still, for employees to do the work and stay involved, hospital leadership had to make a visible commitment and demonstrate that "this lean thing" was serious and was not just the next "initiative de jour." The strategy for supporting lean adoption was multifaceted. The executive team learned that culture change takes time and constant attention. Hospital leaders made it a point to work the improvement agenda into daily routines and support staff knew that time scheduled for lean could not be cancelled for some other meeting or event.

Real estate is power on a hospital campus, so the development of dedicated space for lean staff and team events sent a clear message that this new approach was important to the executives. In fact, renovations enabled new rooms and offices to be built strategically around the corner from the executive suite. Although not everyone will have space available to be set aside for lean activities, we found it invaluable to the development of a high-volume, fast-paced approach to events and training. The space was centrally located and easy to access; leaders, managers, and staff could easily stop by for a chat, a question, or status reports or to drop into an improvement event.

Another strategy the hospital leadership used to support lean activities was to publicize the RIE "report outs" that took place at the end of each event week. These report outs were held in the auditorium and attracted at least 100 employees on a weekly basis. Those who could not make it to the report outs in person had the option of watching the results of the RIEs on any television set on the hospital's campus. By tuning to Channel 16, employees could view a broadcast of the report out. Senior staff members were always in the audience, a seemingly simple but important way of demonstrating that executives valued the opportunity to learn what teams had accomplished that week and to celebrate their successes.

Senior leaders also went beyond just a visible presence. To ensure their support reached the frontline staff, they shared support and administrative responsibility with middle management. Participation in RIEs became mandatory for all managers and all senior leaders had to be a part of at least one event each year.[1] In the second year of the rollout, the hospital took this a step further and incorporated lean participation into the evaluation process. The expectations for involvement with lean varied across staff levels. For instance, department heads had to solve two problems within their unit using A3 thinking and attend at least one RIE report out each year.

Not everyone agreed with using lean to change how the hospital delivered patient care. Some middle managers rightfully felt the process was contrary to the command and control management style that had gotten them to their positions in the first place. Many supervisors had to relinquish the skills they came to see as most valuable in managing staff, including crisis management, solving problems as opposed to enabling staff to solve problems, and dictating action instead of coaching staff; this was a challenging and intimidating task (see Box 2.2).

Required involvement in lean helped alleviate many of the concerns among most managers. Others received additional support, personal coaching, and education. When the executive team felt that it had done as much as it could do to work with an uncooperative manager with no success, that person was counseled and in some cases, ultimately, let go. This action sent a strong message to other middle managers and the rest of the staff.[2]

Box 2.2 **A Contrast in Management Styles**	
TRADITIONAL MANAGEMENT	LEAN THINKING
• Batch and queue production	• One by one, continuous flow
• Functional silos	• Value stream management
• Productivity pushed by targets	• Demand pulled by customer
• Efficiency of the parts	• Throughput focus
• Quality control functions external to process	• Quality checks built into the process in real time
• Specialization • Job descriptions and variation in processes	• Cross functional teams, tightly connected • Shared skills, cross training and standard work
• Review of reports, need to know approach to information	• Visual management, transparency

Source: Adapted from Lean Awareness Training, Simpler Business System©, 2010. Used with permission.

Executives learned that they had to shift their leadership styles as well, realizing that the traditional top-down approach to leadership is not consistent with lean principles. Instead, leaders must assume the role of stating the vision and guiding staff toward it—clearly defining the end goal and enabling staff to define how that goal would be reached. In lean, we aspire to develop stakeholders, problem solvers, and leaders at every level of the organization. This can be very challenging. Bohmer's (2012) work has focused on medical leadership:

> Do we see leadership primarily in terms of change ('transformative' leadership), looking for medical leaders to take existing systems through painful and contentious change? Or do we see medical leadership as an essential component of any programme to assure the performance of existing organisations?

In this book, we discuss the need to establish the standardized processes and support systems necessary to ensure evidence-based practice is being delivered and can be reliably sustained; examples of the application of these are included in Chapters 5 through 9. We continue to explore the elements of leadership that are effective for us and that are effective and appropriate in different situations. A deeper analysis of what current medical leaders are challenged to do can best be summarized as three different roles. Bohmer (2012) describes the first role as addressing the best known way to deliver care in repeatable care situations. Here the leader's focus is on building a system to deliver a known practice and this requires working knowledge of the clinical practice in question by the leader. The second role as described by Bohmer (2012) is to help a diverse team build consensus regarding what is valuable for their patients. Here a leader's focus is the team caring for their patients and helping the team determine value through the eyes of their patients. Leaders caring for teams require deep interpersonal understanding of teams and their dynamics. Finally, the third role for a leader is to create a space for experimentation. Leaders in this role must *lead learning* and celebrate the process of experimentation. In some situations, such as a unit chief or head nurse, a leader may need only to fulfill one of these roles to be successful. In other situations, a single leader may need to fulfill all of these roles.

Learning a new way is humbling. Humility is the first challenge in a lean journey and although leaders may think they are ready it is never a linear path. Lean appears to be, on the surface, a straightforward change model; however, the deeper one digs, the more complicated it can become as it is a *business improvement system* with far-reaching power to transform. It is not easy to both learn a whole new way of operating and lead at the same time.

Senior leaders will learn that lean requires a *paradigm shift* for the entire organization. It may be helpful to start with these key questions: What assessment tools would help my organization begin such an effort? What are my organization's practices? Past ability to sustain changes? Past attempts to change culture? How might my senior cabinet, middle managers, and line staff react to a new way?

Lean helps leaders move away from a reactive state to a proactive state of management. Leaders move from working from the "gut" to working with data. The use of data and being proactive in planning and solving is a radical shift. The key to understanding how to implement lean in health care successfully is to realize that lean leadership is an integral part of lean. At first lean feels like (and, in fact, is) one more thing to do—an "add on." It takes time for leaders to understand the degree to which their own leadership behaviors will need to change—from solving problems to enabling others to do so, from telling direct reports "how to" to coaching them toward defined endpoints but trusting them to be able to figure out how to get there. Leadership of this type cannot be delegated; the literature, specific to lean or more generalizable, is clear about the need for visibility and clarity on the part of the top leader of an organization in order to create change and spark innovation. Without active leadership efforts to change the culture long held behaviors will fail.[3] Leaders within HHC participate in at least one rapid improvement event a year—there is no more definitive statement of commitment to lean than a senior leader of the corporation standing at the wall mapping processes, running experiments in the gemba and struggling to draft standard work with a team of individuals who, at least for the week, "leave their titles at the door."[4]

According to Transformational Leadership theory, introduced by Burns as "Transforming Leadership" and expanded and modified to its present coinage by Bass, a leader's approach can significantly influence the lives of people and organizations. Transformational leaders lead by example, challenge workers to innovate to the point of changing the environment, and achieve organizational change through inspiring and coaching workers. Anyone who has been at a large lean conference has experienced the unique phenomenon of being surrounded by lean practitioners who are at once highly experienced and senior in their field yet are quintessentially humble, unrestrained in sharing their knowledge, and have a cadre of mentees in their wake.[5]

At HHC, hospital executives had to become visible advocates of lean and be strategic about moving out of meetings and into the gemba to "go see, ask why, show respect."[6] Senior leaders were no longer just administrators; they had to be motivators. The combination of these strategies not only contributed to the improvement of patient care but also strengthened the relationships among staff members at all levels of the facility.

Notes

1. Rapid Improvement Events are defined further in Chapter 1. These are 4.5-day, interdisciplinary team-based improvement activities, during which problems are defined, current and target states are mapped, and solutions are generated, tested, and put in place.
2. Coaching is a skill and, as such, takes practice and time. *Managing to Learn* (John Shook, Lean Enterprise Institute, 2008) is a practical guide to leading by asking questions and coaching from the student and the supervisor's perspectives.
3. Kotter, John P. *Leading Change*. Cambridge, MA: Harvard Business Review Press, 1996.
4. Byrne, Art. *The Lean Turnaround: How Business Leaders Use Lean Principles to Create Value and Transform Their Company*. New York: The McGraw-Hill Companies, 2013.
5. Bass, Bernard M., Ronald E. Riggio. *Transformational Leadership*, 2nd ed. Mahwah, NJ: Lawrence Erlbaum Associates, Inc. 2006.
6. John Shook, *CEO of the Lean Enterprise Institute, quoting Fujio Cho, Chairman of Toyota, in the foreword to Gemba Walks* (Jim Womack, Lean Enterprise Institute, 2011).

3

Lean, Safety, and Quality

ROBERT BERDING, RENUKA ANANTHAMOORTHY,

AND LORA GIACOMONI

All too often a major culture shift within an organization is preceded by a criti-cal event that serves as the impetus for necessary changes. Such was the case for Kings County Hospital Center (KCHC) Behavioral Health Services (BHS). BHS had a reputation in the local community as a scary place to be hospitalized, and its lurid-looking "G" building didn't help (see Figure 3.1). If anyone in the local com-munity acted strangely, they were stigmatized as candidates for "G"; the New York Daily News described the building as "modern-day Brooklyn Bedlam." Built in the first half of the twentieth century, it loomed ominously in central Brooklyn with ancient, barred windows and a stark façade. Inside, institutional green paint, the absence of any décor and doors that were locked with skeleton keys confirmed the perception the exterior promised.

A class action lawsuit alleging concerns about quality and safety was brought against the hospital in 2007 by a statewide advocacy group. The United States Department of Justice (DOJ) became involved, began to conduct its own investiga-tion into the service, and, ultimately, imposed a settlement agreement that required extensive remediation by the hospital. Then, in mid-2008, in the midst of settlement discussions with the advocacy group's investigation and ongoing oversight by the DOJ, a patient tragically died while waiting in the psychiatric emergency room. This event garnered worldwide media attention and greatly increased the level of over-sight and demand for change by the DOJ.

Both the plaintiffs' and DOJ investigations produced significant findings that ultimately required extensive corrective actions, and both resulted in court-ordered settlement agreements. The timing and circumstances were ripe for changing the paradigm in BHS. Even those who routinely failed to question current practices and were inclined to resist change were suddenly forced to be open to new possibilities.

The challenge was to how to adopt and apply lean principles[1] in a Behavioral Health setting so as to promote quality and safety. Because the concept is one of

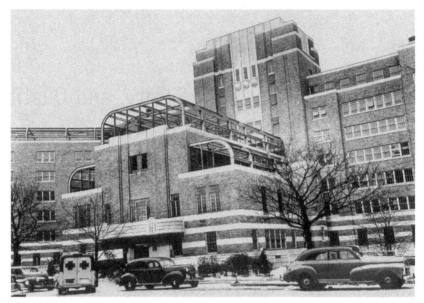

Figure 3.1 "G" Building.

transformation, there was no predefined, cookie-cutter formula for success. Rather, the process we chose first required a commitment to embrace the following five lean principles: (1) The Customer Defines Value; (2) Deliver Value to the Customer Upon Demand; (3) Mutual Respect and Shared Responsibility; (4) Standardize and Solve to Improve; and; (5) Transformational Learning. This "embracing" cannot be expected to occur overnight or result simply from some well-intentioned educational orientation. Rather, these principles must be woven into all quality improvement efforts and reinforced through explicit reminders that tie a specific change to a specific principle.

With this framework in place, it becomes possible to consider past problems in a new light and hypothesize about targeted solutions that can be tested through experimentation. We developed some guiding principles for safety and quality initiatives were conceived:

- Patients, staff, and other stakeholders should feel safer on the units.
- Patient dignity and respect are more readily achieved in an environment that seeks to avoid the use of restraints.
- The voice of the patient needs to become more prominent in the treatment planning process.
- Treatment programs should be more reflective of patients' needs.
- Discharge from inpatient services should be more reflective of the continuum of services available in the community.

One of the first corrective actions taken was a dramatic shoring up of staffing. By the beginning of 2009, many of the BHS staff were new to Kings County Hospital Center, new to each other and new to lean theory and practice. Early decisions had to be made about how to best allocate these new resources. Aside from the obvious need for more direct care providers, it would be necessary to staff and build a robust internal oversight component.

The advocates and DOJ concerns regarding unsafe practices and conditions for mental health patients underscored the inadequacies of quality oversight existing within the BHS. To address these concerns, a dedicated quality management (QM) department was developed to track, trend, and analyze data relating to BHS programs and services. This newly formed department mirrored the established hospital-wide QM structure and included performance improvement (PI), risk management (RM), and regulatory affairs (RA) units, along with the addition of a legal compliance (LC) component. Over time, a data shop (DS) was also added and the department was ultimately renamed BHS Quality and Compliance (Q & C).

Each of these QM units were intended to have distinct responsibilities but would also look at quality and safety issues in a unified fashion. PI quickly established a system for comprehensive, concurrent medical record review and organized projects around such safety issues as assaults and falls. RM performed investigations on all incidents and allegations and kept up with mandatory reporting to relevant external oversight agencies. RA began to organize certification and accreditation processes to ensure appropriate licenses and operating certificates were in place. This was no small task because there were 17 distinct regulatory surveys in 2009 covering the large range of emergency, inpatient, and outpatient services provided throughout central Brooklyn. LC had the responsibility for beginning to address plaintiff and DOJ concerns that flowed from the settlement agreement.

At first, these units met frequently on an ad hoc basis to discuss daily occurrences and how any useful data might be gleaned from the medical record or other sources. There was a good deal of time and effort devoted to attempting to identify potential sources of current data and how to construct more reliable data collection methods. In most instances, there was very little data, in part because of an organizational culture that saw documentation as a means of demonstrating potential culpability related to adverse outcomes. Ironically, many staff did not realize that proper documentation could serve as proof that their actions were "within the scope of Generally Accepted Professional Standards (GAPS)" and therefore it actually provides a measure of protection for them. Rather, there was a widespread belief that if one's name was not in the record, then that person could claim noninvolvement. This was just one of the backward notions that had to be set straight. The fact that 441 surveillance cameras throughout BHS recorded what staff did and did not do did not seem to affect this perception.

KCHC had a long way to go, but it is important to note that although the breadth and depth of problems may not have been fully realized or effectively addressed over time, the need to replace the decrepit G Building had been long recognized. It was near impossible to maintain an encouraging attitude and open dialogue in the somber and depressing old building. Plans to rebuild much of the campus, which poor contained buildings dating to the late 1800s, had been slowly realized over the last several years but had grown ever more conservative as years passed and capital was illusive. Still, after rebuilding the main hospital building, emergency room, ambulatory care center, and surgical services, a new behavioral health building, "R," was rising at the west end of the campus. This building was scheduled to open in January 2009 as the last phase of the hospital's rebuilding plan. It featured large open spaces, abundant light, and modern finishes. The soon-to-be-opened new building devoted to behavioral health care would be larger than many full service hospitals and was, with 266 beds, one of the largest such structures dedicated to acute behavioral health care in the country.

Lean was introduced as "Breakthrough" at the corporate level at roughly the same time as the corrective actions were being developed and applied at KCHC. In late 2008, with the challenge of developing a wholly new approach to behavioral health care at KCHC, corporate leaders offered Breakthrough resources to the hospital to assess existing problems, envision a new future, and develop the infrastructure for the new system of care with a fully integrated improvement structure. However, these resources, in the form of dedicated external sensei (lean experts) and corporate lean staff, were initially greeted with polite skepticism by staff and managers. Having just spent months developing a new, formal quality and compliance structure, was this lean thing going to override local decisions and set the facility back again? How would quality and compliance be integrated with Breakthrough strategies and why was the corporate office asking BHS to dedicate precious local staff to Breakthrough "facilitation and support"? At the end of 2008, with the move to the new R building just 2 months away, lean was first used to review plans for functional adjacencies and patient flow. The process was eye-opening—the new building was beautiful but, absent rational workflows, would soon create staff dissatisfaction that could challenge the level extant in the G building. A series of 5-day rapid improvement events (RIEs) were held in which interdisciplinary teams identified problems and then created, tested and implemented solutions that were celebrated by leadership. These events began to generate enthusiasm and a sense that although the challenges were huge, the team could work together to figure out how to move forward. The learning curve was aided by lean tools such as the DOWNTIME acronym used to reduce operational wastes[2], which are characterized by:

Defects	Transportation
Overproducing	Inventory
Waiting	Motion
Not using skills	Extra-processing

Table 3.1 **Sample Patient Care Quality Improvements Using Lean**

Issue	Before	After
Timeliness of CPEP RN triage	>60 minutes	<20 minutes
Clear Axis I diagnosis	60%	100%
First appointment kept	40%	95%

When this tool was used to successfully plan for and move approximately 200 patients from the G to R buildings over the course of 24 hours with no harm and a minimum of care disruption, staff engagement in lean grew.

It would still take about 2 years before a true synergy developed between the staff and processes utilized for Breakthrough and quality and compliance. The ultimate goal of going beyond traditional definitions of quality and weaving Breakthrough into everyday practice was still a distant vision. Yet, we recognized that there had to be a system that ensured the integrity of the data, which could then be used to set benchmarks and be presented to staff for action. Because Breakthrough and BHS QM had been established on parallel tracks, the early events intertwined both. Staff sought methods to share resources to optimize the opportunities to achieve the desired results. Breakthrough immediately tapped into QM's emerging data capabilities to set quantifiable baselines for selected projects. One of the first RIEs examined patient flow through the psychiatric emergency room. The facilitators and team were skilled at managing individual patient care but unequipped to perform time studies and link key steps to meaningful aggregated data. A QM staffer acted as subject matter expert and worked with the RIE teams to design measurable indicators with thresholds derived from the time studies that could be used to monitor future performance improvement. Conversely, QM emphasized lean values to motivate and empower line staff. It became evident fairly quickly that lean concepts were powerful and could be used to operationalize the needed changes (see Table 3.1).

The core values of lean are grouped together and pursued through the concept of "true north" metrics. This catch-phrase is meant to conjure up the navigational reliability associated with following the geodetic north direction that leads straight over the Earth's surface to the North Pole. The true direction to the "top of the Earth" can always be reached by looking up to the guiding northern star, Polaris. This imagery implies that just like navigators can fix a straight and true course to the top of the earth by keeping Polaris in sight, so too can lean followers reach their goals by keeping true north in sight. Of course, lean true north is not a single shining star, but a small cluster that includes stars named Quality, Safety, Human Development, Timeliness, Cost, and Growth and Development. Maintaining a view across these dimensions ensures a balanced effort that won't result in great savings only to see quality suffer, safer services at exorbitant cost, or higher productivity at the expense of staff dignity. Quantifying and keeping these guiding values in sight, change activities can be organized to make incremental progress toward the true north targets. An organization can then plot navigational points that will lead from its current state to its target state.

Although lean was generally introduced as a methodology for performance improvement in all of these dimensions at BHS, the true north[3] metrics of quality and safety represented a natural fit for the newly formed Quality Management (QM) Department. Much early planning centered on how to promote these concepts to staff. This is not meant to imply that the other true north metrics were undervalued by QM. In fact, there were significant improvements in all of these areas that happily coincided with the emphasis on quality and safety.

Of the two, the need for improved safety was the more obvious. It was not unusual for assaults to occur on the inpatient units—especially during evening, night, and weekend shifts when staffing levels were lower than weekdays. In the old "G" culture, these lower staffing levels led to "survival tactics" on the off shifts when staff would spend their time behind secure nursing stations in an effort to avoid personal injury. Increased safety was critical; achieving buy-in for this objective would not be difficult if quality management could show the correlation between lean projects and decreased personal injuries.

The notion of quality, on the other hand, was an abstract concept for most staff. Although there had been many advances in behavioral health science over the past decades, Kings County had not kept pace. The level of care could be compared to the large state institutions of the late 1970s when the clunky transition from custodial care to psychiatric treatment was still in its early stages. Staff attitudes toward patients were often paternalistic, where good behavior was rewarded with discharge and other behaviors were met with medication or physical restraints. Although staff recognized that these practices contributed to creating a revolving door for the majority of patients, there was little insight within the organization about how to change. Therefore, the notion of quality was introduced incrementally and was accompanied by enhanced patient engagement and a move to the patient-centered recovery model of care.

Addressing Quality and Safety

The first question was, "Where to start?" Based on the DOJ findings and class action allegations that both quality and safety were lacking, this would prove to be no easy task. It seemed logical to enter at the same point that the patient would arrive: through the Comprehensive Psychiatric Emergency Program—Emergency Room (CPEP-ER).

While still planning the first RIE for this area, lean thinking was at first informally put into motion through quality management. The CPEP-ER was a crowded space full of people. In addition to patients and providers, the presence of family members, friends, patient advocates, and aides made it difficult to account for everyone in the CPEP-ER at any given point in time. An elemental tracking process launched a short time earlier attempted to redress this, but it had quickly been limited by the dearth of any relevant and reliable data system. Data collection was manually collected by staff who completed handwritten logs about all the goings-on in the CPEP-ER.

These "trackers" scurried around the CPEP-ER making paper notations on arrival times, stages of evaluation, dispositions, and most everything in between. Often, they would use hand signals across the crowded room to indicate which patient and/or process each was tracking at the moment so as not to duplicate efforts. At the end of each shift, the trackers would dutifully submit their stack of paper notations for data entry by other clerical staff. Observations were tallied, and a weekly summary of the recorded events was produced.

In keeping with the lean spirit, the trackers were engaged in discussions about CPEP-ER processes to gain their perspective. As objective observers of the grass roots process, the trackers had a wealth of knowledge and useful insights about waste in the system. It was apparent to the trackers that although established procedures existed, there was no true standard work in the CPEP-ER. Although most staff members were well intentioned, some were more efficient and thorough than others in carrying out assigned duties. For example, some nurses were routinely able to begin the initial nursing care assessment within 30 minutes of patient arrival, whereas others only achieved this timeliness benchmark on an intermittent basis. This reinforced the lean value that those more efficient and thorough providers could and would blaze trails of improvement if allowed an opportunity to do so. The task became to identify internal best practices and develop standards of work that could be benchmarked as quality indicators. Eventually, this approach would be used to drive practice and eliminate the workplace variability that was at the root of BHS' inefficiency.

Gaps in the process of discharging patients from the CPEP-ER, including documentation of discharge information, posed additional challenges. Discharge information was to be collected in the Electronic Health Record (EHR). The EHR was the preferred primary source of data, but retrieving anything meaningful required the elimination of Garbage In, Garbage Out (GIGO). Early attempts identified an abundance of Nothing In, Nothing Out (NINO). This was especially true in electronically documenting discharge dates and times from the CPEP-ER. The first report showed about a 50% compliance rate for entering this data into the EHR.

Providers were canvassed for their opinion on this phenomenon. Some believed the paper log was the official documentation site for this information. Others thought that the Situation-Background-Assessment-Recommendation (SBAR) Handoff was sufficient for communicating the event. The SBAR is in fact a comprehensive technique for coordinating critical information that requires immediate attention and action concerning a patient's condition. The Situation represents what is going on at the moment with the patient (I observed Mr. A pacing rapidly in CPEP-ER). The Background contextualizes the situation (Mr. A has a diagnosis of paranoid schizophrenia, history of assaultive behavior when becoming agitated, and has been waiting for 3 hours to be transferred to the inpatient unit). Assessment anticipates that the staff member will offer an opinion on what the problem might be (Mr. A appears to be growing increasingly agitated by the long waiting period). Finally, the expectation is that a Recommendation will be made (Mr. A should be safely escorted to the inpatient unit now and reassured that he will be well cared for). However, as good as SBAR is for attending to the needs of the patient at the moment, it is meaningless for data collection unless someone records the events in the prescribed data entry fields.

Some staff were completely unaware that such a data field existed in the electronic health record. Clearly, some standard work and staff education were needed on this topic. Without this type of data entry, it would be impossible to monitor quality indicators such as overall wait time from CPEP-ER to Inpatient Services or safety indicators like overcrowding.

Using lean thinking, the CPEP-ER team gathered and drew up the process on a display board. The waste stared back at the group as the numerous, overlapping steps were listed on the board: duplicate data entry fields for physicians and nurses; duplicate electronic and paper data entry requirements; redundant hand-off processes; and no standard for documenting an official discharge date and time.

After the RIE, staff satisfaction was bolstered by a new QM visual management report that showed RN discharge data entry was now occurring at a 95% rate, or nearly double the rate of the original reports. In addition, QM began to publish the "success rates" for nurses who performed this task. Nurses with high rates of

---

Lessons Learned

Staff generally react favorably to visual management tools and are inclined to take immediate action when presented with obvious opportunities for improvement. It did not take long to agree on and implement a more efficient model. In "just do it" fashion, the RN discharge form was designated as the official site for documenting discharge date and time while other sites were eventually eliminated. This pleased the team, in part because it eliminated some unnecessary steps from their daily routine and equally because their voice was instrumental in effectuating change.

appropriate discharge data entry were acknowledged at rounds and team meetings for a job well done. At the same time, nurses with lower compliance rates were not chastised or penalized in any manner. Rather, all such instances were treated as "education opportunities" and individualized instruction and reinforcement was provided until the nurse was completely competent to complete the task on a consistent basis.

A successful formula began to emerge from the lean philosophy. Begin by engaging and inviting participation from each team member to improve quality and safety. Be sure to take small steps on the way toward reaching eventual long-term goals. Each step would be a building block to the next step. Each building block would be fashioned by the input of the person who was responsible for the task.

The approach was simple in concept but, as is usually the case in real life, difficult in implementation. There were to be occasions of conflicting priorities, battling egos, lackluster motivation, and plain old poor planning. In retrospect, the most daunting barrier was the failure of all staff to embrace lean early on and establish its role in the mainstream of daily caregiving rather than relegating it to some ancillary function. Most staff who served in BHS, however, bought into lean and, with group energy and perseverance, strove for optimal results. Gradually, the culture was changing.

It was also a fortunate circumstance that the introduction of lean coincided with a move from the infamous "G" building to the new "R" building (see Figure 3.2). It was as bright as the former had been such a contrast of bleak. It was a perfect setting for incubating new lean ideas. It was as if the despair associated with the old building had been left behind, and everyone, staff and patients alike, was excited about the possibilities of a new beginning.

More importantly, this set the tone for quality management. This was not going to be another top-down, shame-blame, administrative silo of meaningless data collection and reports. Not only was staff input sought after, each person's contribution was valued and considered as vital paving stones being laid on the road to improvement. These stones were gathered in a variety of ways. The most common method was through one-to-one dialogue in the person's assigned work area. Rather than causing dread by asking staff to appear in front of a conference room full of frowning supervisors, a single QM manager would wander down to a unit with some data in hand. The QM manager would introduce him or herself and explain the purpose of the visit, which was to gain some insight about the data. The staff member was asked to hypothesize about how the current conditions came about and offer suggestions on potential improvements. These collegial dialogues always had follow-up visits to discuss any progress or barriers to success. Over time, many staff began to seek out QM staff to proactively offer their paving stones of wisdom and insight.

It was also important that the QM tone mirrored that of other corporate initiatives. Just Culture[4] espoused principles for achieving a culture in which frontline

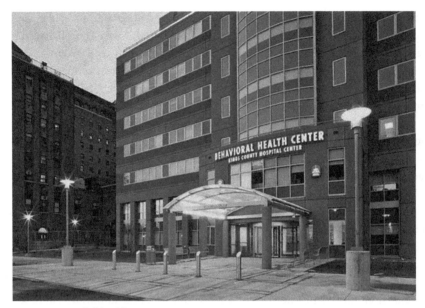

Figure 3.2 New "R" building.

personnel felt comfortable disclosing errors—including their own—while main-taining professional accountability. TeamSTEPPS[5] sought to improve team struc-tures, individual leadership skills, situation monitoring, mutual support, and clear communication. Essential for our success, there was an obvious and strong corpo-rate commitment to setting a tone for cooperation, communication, accountability, and continuous improvement.

However, this informal beginning would need to be rapidly cultivated and intro-duced to much larger numbers of staff. As helpful and necessary as the trackers were in establishing a data collection process, the long-term solution needed to be more automated and robust. A project to identify the data that clinical leadership and line staff needed to manage for daily improvement and yield quantitative performance measures was also initiated at the same time.

The First Rapid Improvement Event

The next step was to directly engage the providers in a formal RIE. Given the orga-nizational history, this would be no small feat. There were healthy and proven atti-tudes of suspicion and distrust for administration, especially a new one. There was no tradition of staff participation in the improvement process, only negative reper-cussions if found to be at fault for any adverse outcome. Therefore, buy-in and cul-ture change could not be achieved through mere promises of incentives; it had to be earned by demonstrating its actual benefit to participating staff members.

We chose to start off simple and show providers that data could be used to highlight their accomplishments and how their efforts translated into improved quality and safety. Producing data that would be relevant and meaningful to clinicians was the next course of action. For this RIE, the focus would be on the quality of the intake process.

Inconsistencies in the intake process frequently caused patient flow bottlenecks in the CPEP-ER. A bottleneck creates a capacity limitation and does not allow the system to meet the demand of the customer.

Data associated with the process was shared with staff and it was immediately apparent that inefficiencies caused problems for everyone. There were instances when assessments were duplicated for some patients and missed for others because there was no standard work for assigning patients upon arrival. Another problem was that some patients would be "handed off" between shifts but wait for services as additional new patients entered the area. It was also evident that some staff completed the bulk of the assessments, whereas others produced very little documentation. Ultimately, all staff were frustrated because they felt bogged down in a ceaseless intake cycle and patients were disgruntled because of unnecessarily long wait times.

All aspects of the process were examined by the team. The solution approach to this problem was to establish work standards that could be easily understood and carried out by assigned staff. This early workflow included a role for Hospital Police (HP) to log CPEP-ER patients and ensure that no contraband was brought into the facility (this role was later relegated to specially trained behavioral health aides). The standard work for HP was depicted through a visual management tool similar to the one below by listing step-by-step instructions along with scripted responses for routine patient encounters (see Figure 3.3).

These visual management tools made it simple for everyone to understand their role and the roles of others. Another benefit was that these simple steps could be easily monitored and used to create reports about the effectiveness of the process. Most clinicians were glad to receive these reports because it validated their concerns and highlighted the need for a more organized approach to change. This was especially true for staff whose production level was proven to be higher than others.

A follow-up RIE was devoted to the monitoring process for critical indices related to the various elements of patient care in the CPEP-ER. During this event it was identified that the current data collection method was person powered and labor intensive. Disparate data sources often produced conflicting quantitative reports, and information was not communicated to the clinical staff in real time. Through a series of rapid experiments, we were able to identify various ways in which technology could be used to reduce the preparation time of reports. This, coupled with other efficiencies implemented in QM, allowed staff to focus more on performance improvement activities rather than chasing data.

The CPEP-ER was the primary focus of the plaintiff settlement agreement. As such, with lean-focused improvements and outcome data, BHS began to establish a

1) *Keep the patient calm. Go by the script HP1a.*
2) *Ensure you have logged the patient into the Patient Log Book.*
3) *Ensure the visitors do not bring any contraband into CPEP-ER.*

1) *Keep the patient calm and follow script.*

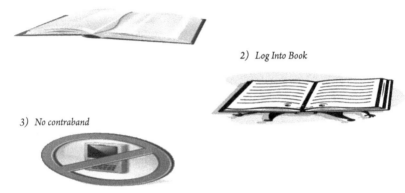

2) *Log Into Book*

3) *No contraband*

Figure 3.3 Hospital police standard work visual management tool.

level of credibility with that group that didn't exist before. The benefits of lean were already yielding some quick victories; improved patient flow, increased staff satisfaction and external trust. Granted, all of these were of very small measure at first, but it was a start and the momentum was beginning to build.

From the initial introduction to lean thinking through the first formal RIE, champions were beginning to emerge from among the rank and file. It was now time to take a step back and begin to plan out the scope and timelines for ongoing implementation, especially to comply with the DOJ settlement agreement.

Incorporating the Voice of the Customer

Staff attention had initially been gained by offering a genuine partnership with, and full recognition of, staff. This was effective in kick-starting the process of improvement but lacked the voice of the persons who ultimately would decide whether the true north metrics were achieved from their perspective. In health care, this is the patient. In lean, this is the customer.

It is an unfortunate reality, but even among behavioral health professionals, there often exists a reluctance to meaningfully consider the perspective of the person receiving services. Even the current terminology, *recipient of care*, implies a passive role for the person who is meant to benefit by the interventions. There is no simple explanation as to why this type of attitude still exists in health care today.

Variables such as cultural beliefs, ignorance of etiology, and common fear contribute to this ongoing, unspoken bias. It is unfathomable that a health care provider would discount or dismiss the input of a person about to have a baby. Yet, many behavioral health staff do not routinely solicit and incorporate the preferences of the person receiving behavioral health services despite regulations that require such a relationship.

Nonetheless, with the changes being made at KCHC, patient views became a nonnegotiable tandem of values when viewed through the lean QM lens. Our goal was to improve service quality and personal safety for persons served, and the success of these improvements would ultimately be evaluated against the satisfaction of the person receiving the service.

Fortunately, most staff adopted a mantra that echoed the sentiment of "Let's do our best for our patients." The value attributed to the contribution of the person served was greatly reinforced through the presence of "peer counselors," former patients hired to engage and advocate for current patients. Even predating the plaintiff and DOJ mandates and recommendations, HHC made a significant investment in hiring ample numbers of peer counselors. Peers provided a unique perspective, compassion, insight, intensity, and, most of all, a strong voice that represented our behavioral health population. Peers are in an advanced stage of recovery and are skilled in the use of appropriate disclosure, role modeling, active listening, and other normalizing interpersonal communication techniques. They embody hope and also had graduated from an intensive peer-training program (i.e., Howie the Harp Advocacy Center in New York).

A peer's role generally includes patient engagement from first presentation in the CPEP through inpatient/outpatient treatment. This encounter involves an orientation to the therapeutic milieu, explanation of schedules, patient rights and unit-based safety procedures along with encouragement to express treatment expectations by taking an active role in the treatment planning process. Beyond this initial meeting, peers will also make themselves available to represent any patient in a treatment team meeting who chooses this level of support. As a patient-designated treatment team representative, the staff rely on the peer to review individual patient goals, provide information about potential resources, offer suggestions based on personal experience, and follow up as needed to promote the successful achievement of goals.

Holding key roles in the BHS improvement process has empowered peers to speak freely in other forums of the organization. For the peers, the respect accorded their opinions in the RIEs demonstrates our sincere concern that we must have their voices on a wide variety of issues. It has also helped to begin to define a truer sense of what it takes for an organization to be patient centered. Prior to participation in RIEs, some peers were perceived, and perhaps believed themselves, that as individuals they were limited to ancillary duties. As long as patients were offered an ear to listen or a rights form to sign, the peer had done his or her job. Now, most

Lessons Learned

One of the most effective ways to empower staff is to cast them into vital roles in the improvement process. It quickly became standard to include peers on RIE teams or just do its (JDIs); 100% of BHS events include input from peers. The peers, in turn, were tenacious in incorporating the feedback from current inpatients. The result is that the inclusion of peers began to establish an identity for the person served by combining the presence of a former inpatient with the views of someone who was currently housed on one of the units.

peers are a commanding presence in team meetings in sharing their observations and perceptions regarding ongoing treatment. There have already been two promotions from among their ranks: the first to a patient care associate (PCA) and a second to community liaison worker. This advancement lent further credibility to the group and served as a reminder that all patients have potentially untapped potential for gainful and meaningful employment. Recovery IS possible!

Peers are able to break through difficult emotional barriers, a poignant example of which relates to a young patient who had experienced the sudden and unexpected death of a loved one only a few short months prior to admission. At first, the patient presented as effusive, positive, friendly, and talkative. This individual was also constantly in motion and unable to sleep. A peer ably engaged the patient by sharing personal experience about effectively dealing with grief. As a result, the individual was then able to grieve freely and returned soon thereafter to home in the community. This type of engagement has repeated itself many times over. Although it is difficult to precisely quantify the impact of lean participation, it is likely that such scenarios would not occur as often without the empowerment that resulted from peer inclusion.

In this regard, KCHC BH has come a long way but still has ample room for further incremental improvement. The treatment team meeting process is still making strides in meaningfully including the patient. Most staff members have accepted the fact that the person served is the most integral member of the treatment team. There is also a healthy respect for the role of other stakeholders, such as family and friends. In lean thinking, this process may need a few more "pass-throughs," whereby work standards newly created through lean are viewed and evaluated through a more sophisticated and mature gap analysis. At the least, the bar has been set at a level that contemplates and values BHS patient participation.

There were a number of "lessons learned" during this process. First, it was shortsighted to attempt to integrate peers into the treatment team process without either a structured team format for information sharing or a standard work to describe their respective roles and responsibilities. Early successes turned on the personalities and tenacity of the individuals who were determined to succeed. Later, best practices emerged through modeling their ingenuity, persuasiveness, and passion, and the opportunities to demonstrate these qualities arose through lean activities—RIEs, JDIs, and educational sessions.

In addition, the process of designating peers as members of the treatment team was not without some unintended tension. Prior to their inclusion as RIE team members, a peer would meet with a patient apart from the team and then "advocate" for the expressed wishes of the patient to the team. Once becoming a team member, there was sometimes pressure to "support" the team's plan made "for" the patient over the desired plan expressed by the patient. In this way, the "advocacy" role may have been compromised in the eyes of the patient, thereby diminishing the level of trust. However, most peers remained sensitive to this potential conflict and were able to effectively balance these occasionally competing roles.

Creating the Master Plan

We established a steering committee to guide the development of organizational goals and accompanying RIEs and other improvement activities. BHS leadership, staff composition, and routines varied greatly in the early steering committee meetings. The enthusiasm level was mostly on the plus side, but the mindsets of the "steerers" were far from unified and cohesive. Perceptions about Breakthrough among the group ranged from extreme buy-in to reluctant acceptance of a forced corporate exercise. This diversity of perception caused stilted discussions during many of the early meetings. Rather than simply focusing on quality and safety planning, there were often distractions concerning which staff members had more pressing assignments and the validity of the RIEs.

On occasion, the skepticism of naysayers appeared justifiable as some RIEs suffered from a variety of shortcomings, such as overreaching goal statements or tenuous sustainment plans. For example, there was a naivety about the ability of the organization to comprehensively solve complex problems in a single event. Perhaps this was fueled by the pressure to fulfill DOJ mandates in an expedient manner or the overexuberance of well-intentioned lean neophytes. Whatever the underlying reasons, in retrospect it was unrealistic to expect we could create sustainable work standards prior to more fully delineating the intricacies of many problems. When dealing with pervasive behavioral health issues such as emergency room patient flow or violence reduction, an organization should expect to perform a series of RIEs that build on the lessons learned from earlier attempts.

Another challenge we faced was that steering committee members were attempting to simultaneously learn about the lean process and operationalize it on the units. This was equivalent to reading instructions about how to operate a motor vehicle while driving a tractor trailer along a busy interstate highway. In short, although the preliminary knowledge was only rudimentary, the task was high pressured and immediate.

The most glaring weakness of the early steering committee is that it did not yet represent the "guiding force" of Behavioral Health. In the beginning, it was an appendage to the department and subservient to competing leadership forums. As such, the methods and outcomes were marginalized as "not officially adopted" and therefore suspect.

Those other leadership forums also ranged in level of authority and scope of participation. There was the widely attended, but largely ineffective, clinical council (later restructured to better integrate Breakthrough and renamed the quality council) that superficially presented and discussed reams of collected data. Essentially, it was a parallel universe that was paralyzed by the abundance of regulatory requirements flowing down from the DOJ settlement agreement. Moreover, although the clinical council was meant to be a performance improvement activity, there was little thought given to how it may fit in with Breakthrough.

Many leaders sat on both the steering committee and quality council but did not recognize the connectedness or inter-relationship between these meetings. This does not mean to impugn the visionary capability of the leaders; in fact, Behavioral Health had assembled a stellar team of leaders with exceptional skills and talents. The lack of early recognition can be attributed to the sheer volume of constant oversight surveys and changing the culture of a large organization that simply did not allow ample time for full analysis of the issues.

Along with the clinical council, there were various other leadership groups such as the top management team (TMT), which was the real driving entity for BHS. It included service and clinical department heads who had divergent views about Breakthrough. There were the zealots who fueled the RIEs, the disinterested who were too consumed with their own responsibilities to consider the value of Breakthrough and the naysayers who were proud not to have "drunk the Kool-Aid." Because the alternate leadership forums had larger and more authoritarian roles in the organization, the steering committee had to begin as a second tier planning venue.

It was not until the completion of the first Value Stream Analysis that the balance of power began to shift. The directive was clear from corporate and hospital executive leaders that Breakthrough was not going to be a fleeting initiative. Using Breakthrough was a mandate and not an option. The emphasis was that quality and safety were to be achieved using lean principles, and all organizational leaders would be evaluated in part on how successful they were in implementing these changes. Thus, the responsibility for setting a visionary course fell squarely on the BHS Steering Committee. The committee was a cross-functional BHS leadership group that set the overall parameters and provided high-level guidance to project leaders. It also had the responsibility for incorporating the viewpoints of all stakeholders and providing advice to process owners, the individuals who "owned" difference processes that were to be improved. The committee then reported up through the Hospital-Wide Executive Steering Committee, a site-level executive leadership group responsible for all improvement work occurring across the hospital campus. Lean was working, based on the upward trends of RIE metrics. For example, the RN triage time had been reduced from more than 60 minutes to less than 20 minutes.

Lean Meets the Department of Justice

These successes spurred BHS to employ lean thinking to all the provisions of the DOJ settlement agreement by establishing "workgroups" for each major section. Each workgroup was to use A3 thinking, especially in analyzing and closing gaps between the current and target states. This problem-solving technique promoted consensus building among workgroup members, thereby unifying their efforts to create simple, systematic methodologies that would evolve into new work standards. This did not mean that all the naysayers were yet convinced, but the tide had become too forceful to outwardly battle against the inevitable. If it was not possible to have unanimous personal buy-in of all stakeholders at this time, then at least everyone was willing to row in the same direction and express optimism about eventual success.

Workgroup Approach

There were 13 workgroups in all, consisting of Treatment Planning, Restrictive Interventions, Quality Assurance, Environment of Care, Assessment, Behavior Management, Pharmacy, Programming, Medical/Nursing, Information Technology, Training, Practice Guidelines and Discharge/Aftercare. Each had a process owner who took on the ultimate responsibility for realizing objectives that were measured by key process indicators. The process owners had authority to make any changes that RIE teams developed. The process owner was supported by co-team leaders who organized and directed workgroup functions. The number of groups and group members naturally led to very wide participation and integration of workgroup activities.

These workgroups were at first conceptualized as "building blocks." Each group would have multidisciplinary representation consisting of staff who had demonstrated some level of expertise, interest, and/or other specialized knowledge. The charge was to make a careful study of known best practices in each area, formulate a plan that optimally fit the needs of BHS patients, and present the model back to the steering committee for ultimate approval and implementation. The groups were expected to meet at least once a week in between other regularly scheduled assignments. The meetings were to be brief in nature, meant only to assign individual tasks and provide updates on progress and assist with the removal of impediments to foster continuous, forward movement.

The large workgroup structure was necessary because the DOJ settlement agreement was a massive document with hundreds of stipulations that required strict compliance. Obviously, not all stipulations could be addressed equally from the outset so priorities were set within each workgroup. For example, the Assessment workgroup was led by the adult inpatient chief of service, the process owner, along with a pediatric inpatient psychologist and assistant director of social work as co-team leaders. In addition, the workgroup included representation from other disciplines such as nursing, therapeutic rehabilitation, and peers. Rather than working within their customary "discipline silos" to resolve aspects of problems germane to that group, members began to expand their thinking and examine potential root causes.

Among the quality council's highest priorities was a major reworking of all risk assessment tools. The workgroup diligently followed the A3 model and created numerous process maps as a visual representation of the sequential flow of the process. Recall that the A3 model is designed to take a workgroup through the following steps: (1) Reason For Action; (2) Initial State; (3) Target State; (4) Gap Analysis; (5) Solution Approach; (6) Rapid Experiments; (7) Completion Plan; (8) Confirmed State; and (9) Insights.

Essentially, A3 provides a useful structure for managing all daily activities. It is so named because it requires being printed out on the large A3 size paper that is necessary to visually capture all of this information on one side of a single sheet. Some of the steps are self-evident, whereas others employ hierarchical tools to arrive at conclusions. The first three steps can be relatively easier to articulate because there is a defined problem in the present state.

Most staff working on RIEs move quickly through this part, but it is important to get these three "boxes" right; if the problem statement, or reason for action, isn't clear, then everything that flows from it will likely be off-base or similarly murky. The gap between initial and target states, represented in "box 4," seeks to identify the root cause of the defined problem(s) and usually presents some challenges because it is hard to simply imagine ways to arrive at a target state using

---

Lessons Learned

A3 thinking can be used consistently within the organization to promote shared thinking processes and similar outcomes-based expectations among staff.

only abstract logic, and we are often tempted at this stage to simply "solve" the problem before fully understanding it. Rather, we use the "5 Whys" technique (ask "why?" five times) as well as fishbone diagrams and data. The 5 Whys are useful for drilling down to the root cause of an issue. This exercise begins by proposing a superficial answer to the problem and then continues to delve to deeper layers of cause by asking "Why?" for each successive proposed answer. Eventually, the group needs to decide what the "deep" root cause is and propose solutions to address it. The process shifts from the theoretical to the practical as the rapid experiments are conceived and tested in the workplace. As the RIE week winds down, the RIE team is charged with completing the fundamental task of defining achievable completion plans that will be confirmed with hard data metrics measuring true north values.

The nine steps, or boxes, of the A3 flow logically one to the next and provide a framework for thinking through an issue from the original problem point to its proven solution. For example, it was identified that some parts of the risk assessment were incorporated into the initial nursing assessment whereas other more specialized risk assessments were triggered by the answers to certain general assessment responses. This process came to light through use of the A3 and was easily remedied by the creation of a single combined risk assessment tool.

Assessment Workgroup

Some workgroups had longer lists of deliverables than others. For example, there was a DOJ requirement for the establishment of High Risk Assessments for the inpatient units and psychiatric emergency room. For the Project workgroup to undertake a task of this magnitude, it was necessary to convene a variety of disciplines for a significant period of time. Although the workgroup was able to complete some preliminary investigation on the subject, there was simply not enough time for them to see the task through to a proper completion.

To resolve this time allocation problem, it was decided that a slightly expanded but intensive specialty group would be formed to properly study the assessment issues and make recommendations. Thus, an RIE was conducted to review the range of High Risk Assessments and the tools utilized to determine the amount of risk.

This RIE Assessment Team consisted of some Assessment workgroup members plus some key unit staff who were responsible for completion of assessments. Four and a half days was allotted for the RIE, which represents the established standard for all such Breakthrough events.

The early part of the week proceeded in rapid fashion. The Reason for Action was clearly defined because an ineffectual assessment process impacted quality and safety. By the end of the second day, the group had completed a very insightful Gap Analysis between the current and target states. The third day was mostly devoted to rapid experiments where team members go to the workplace to try out some of the concepts discussed during the Gap Analysis. The fourth day is used to analyze results of the rapid experiments, solidify the solution approach, formulate a completion plan, and identify a confirmed state that included data elements to be used as performance threshold measures when later assessing progress toward the confirmed state. Finally, on Friday the RIE workgroup presented their findings to the whole organization to recognize and celebrate success and field any questions about the process and upcoming implementation plans.

The RIE process turned out to be a highly successful strategy because it allowed sufficient time for the task and incorporated the expertise of more staff who would perform the assessments. In fact, it then became commonplace for the Project workgroups to complete their assigned tasks through a corresponding RIE.

Over time, the assessment workgroup performed an extensive literature search and created new policies for risk of suicide, self-harm, violence, elopement, and falls. What was new for the organization was that it represented the first time that policy development was coming straight out of the people actually doing the work through the RIE process. Prior to this time, RIEs had been used almost exclusively to promote new work standards, but the actual policies had remained part of the other leadership forums. Although still having to be vetted through the TMT, the self-harm policies were a direct result of an RIE.

Policy Revision

The fact that policy change could come from an RIE further reinforced the pride and ownership of RIE team members. As time went on, RIEs continued to support a shift away from leaders directing RIEs, which had been necessary to get through early resistance and set the pace of improvement activity. The RIE process set the tone that all team members' contributions were important and could rise to the level of written rules that would be used by all staff. Of course, this shift change was accompanied by some substantial challenges. Studies have shown that health care providers who are more satisfied with their work environment are less likely to seek employment elsewhere.[6]

As the details and policies of more and more changes were documented, version control also became a nightmare. For example, an RIE might have created new standard work based on the findings of a rapid experiment. That policy might have been tweaked by the TMT. Then, DOJ may have opined and recommended some changes. After that, the workgroup may have had suggested modifications based on lessons learned from more extensive field use. Even worse, some of these recommendations and suggestions may have been in conflict with each other. It became extremely confusing at times trying to determine which modifications to ultimately adopt and which version contained the agreed-upon language.

Many prior policies had come about through the hard labor of others who did not participate in the RIE. Or, some staff members who had a special interest in a project were not selected for the workgroup. This caused some amount of resentment at times, which surfaced as criticism of the RIE outcomes. This phenomenon lessened as more staff had opportunities to serve as workgroup members, but it still lingers among small pockets of the organization. The need to include and incorporate all members of the organization is one reason why the concept of spread is so important.

The assessment workgroup pioneered significant developments by identifying true north metrics for safety and developing the pathways to achieving specific targets. The scope of high risk assessments included suicide, self-harm, assault, sexual aggression (predator and victim), elopement, and falls. Previously, these individual risk assessments had been either lumped together (suicide and self-harm) or considered mutually exclusive of one another (sexual aggression and elopement). Now, the patient was being considered in totality, and prevention became the focus instead of reactionary stop-gap measures (STAT medications, 1:1 use and/or restraints). Measures, such as restraint rates, IM usage rates, and recidivism rates, began to be effectively tracked and trended and the data were used to make further improvements.

In some ways, the workgroup concept was powerful because it brought different disciplines and backgrounds to the table in search of sustainable solutions to long-standing problems. On the other hand, the logistics of scheduling and fully staffing all the workgroups proved challenging to the organization's "heijunka," or load balancing. There was an ongoing strain on the number of members needed to meet the volume of work required of each group. In addition, the flow, or progressive achievement of tasks, was somewhat stilted because of a natural dependency of some tasks on pre-occurring events. For example, the Treatment Planning workgroup would be limited in planning work standards until a clear picture emerged to delineate the Assessment and Reassessment processes.

Nonetheless, the workgroups made formidable strides in all areas. Of particular note, the Programming workgroup conceptualized and implemented a dynamic pairing of creative arts therapists and patient advocates that was able to offer qualitative programming designed to be part of a treatment regimen instead of merely recreational distractions.

Practice Guideline Workgroup

Another qualitative improvement came about from the efforts of the Practice Guideline workgroup. Up until this point, there had been great variability in diagnosing the patient population. It would not be unusual for a patient to have a wide variety of diagnoses over a period of years because the prevailing practice was to ignore prior history and provide a "de jour" diagnosis based on whatever psychiatric symptomology was being presented at the moment. Early qualitative reviews raised concerns about the number of patients who were diagnosed as Schizophrenia Not Otherwise Specified (NOS) despite having well-documented histories of diagnosable mental illness. Once again, a workgroup, this time the Project workgroup, collaborated with an RIE team to produce a final product that improved quality and safety in the diagnostic process. Baseline research was conducted by the workgroup leading up to the RIE. The event itself produced a time-sensitive enhancement to the electronic health record, which forced clinicians to resolve an NOS diagnosis (see Table 3.1) in a timely manner. In addition, it produced three distinct diagnostic algorithms for (1) schizophrenia; (2) depression; and (3) bipolar disorder.

The NOS diagnosis soon became synonymous with "no diagnosis." The Practice Guideline workgroup was charged with eradicating this practice. This was accomplished by instituting diagnostic algorithms based on published best practices such as the American Psychiatric Association Diagnostic and Statistical Manual of Mental Disorders, American Academy of Child and Adolescent Psychiatry Practice Parameters, Texas Medication Algorithm Project Procedural Manual, and New York City Health and Hospitals Corporation practice guidelines. This approach was severely challenged by many physicians in the beginning, but the workgroup members were extremely thorough in their research and thoughtful in educating physicians on the benefits of establishing an accurate diagnosis that would guide treatment over the lifetime of the patient.

These examples give insights into the value and effectiveness of using A3 thinking in all facets of organizational change. However, change cannot occur simply in the "laboratory" of a workgroup and must be proven in field testing.

Early Attempts at Training

Now that the steering committee and workgroups were in place, the next concern was how to teach staff all of the new policies and procedures in a comprehensive yet efficient manner that were put in place together with the many standards of work and treatment algorithms that had been developed. The sheer volume of needed training would require a daunting number of hours.

The first thought was to continue with the traditional BHS model of discipline—specific training. In this way, discipline supervisors would provide the needed training for subordinate staff. However, this seemed counterintuitive to the emerging team-building model and was eventually rejected as a viable option.

An RIE was then held on the topic of training. It was facilitated by a physician team leader. It produced a very effective standard work for training on the topic of non-crisis intervention. Despite the early effectiveness of this approach, it was not able to be sustained primarily because of the difficulties in scheduling physicians to participate in the process. Eventually, over the next year all physicians received the training through a combination of classroom and unit-based training sessions.

Next we attempted to capitalize on an existing, successful model. The Nursing Department routinely held extensive training for nursing staff. It was thought that the nursing educators could teach expanded curriculums for all staff. Again, like with the disciple specific model, there was a lack of cohesiveness, and team building remained a challenge.

Finally, in a much later stage of development, training fell under a revamped quality council process where the unit leader took on the responsibility for training unit staff. This information was added to the monthly quality reports and woven into the ongoing projects for each unit. The further correlation between staff training and demonstrated competency is discussed later in this section under "Moving From a Top-Down Model to a Hub and Spokes Model."

Taking It to the Gemba

The next step was to test the new workgroup theories and propose practices on "pilot units." In lean speak, this was taking it to the "gemba," or the place where the actual work is done. This is where the services are provided and therapeutic work is done. As a starting point, two such units were chosen as the pilot sites. The choice was based on the skill sets and team functioning of the unit-based interdisciplinary staff, as well as the leadership skills of the unit chief, unit manager, and associate unit chief.

One unit was selected from Adult Inpatient Psychiatry (AIP) and the other from the Child and Adolescent Psychiatry Inpatient Service (CAPIS). These units were the first recipients of the workgroup initiatives. The unit-based staff received intensive training and monitoring via the enhanced methodologies in addition to the customary training and monitoring provided across all service units.

The QM Department, in coordination with the other workgroups, developed the monitoring mechanisms and conducted ongoing regular monitoring across BHS but with special emphasis on the pilot units. After 6 months of full compliance with the enhancements implemented on the pilot units, further plans were developed to roll out the initiatives to other units on an incremental basis.

In essence, the pilot units were a proving ground for the workgroup initiatives. Pilot unit staff were engaged in providing feedback and in fact were responsible for many improvements along the way. A sense of pride and friendly competition began to emerge among the units. Most of these staff were highly engaged and frequently shared observations about the effectiveness of the process. Clearly a new era was emerging from the shadows of the abandoned "G" building. There was an increasing reliance on "genchi gembutsu,"[7] which means "Going to the source to find the facts to make correct decisions, build consensus and achieve goals." In this way, staff gained a thorough understanding of a condition in the workplace by confirming information or data through their personal observations at the source of the condition. For example, staff could analyze data from a remote location and see statistical evidence that restraint usage had decreased on a pilot unit. Further, they could read about the strategies used to successfully achieve that goal. However, it is much more conducive for gaining a fuller appreciation of the accomplishment when walking through the area and observing the nuance of the change. This is when the "conditions" come to life. It is a shallow fact to know that a list of high-risk patients is produced on a daily basis. The utility of that list comes alive when observing how the preparer collects the data, how the information is disseminated to the treatment team, how the team communicates relevant updates and the accompanying esprit de corps that energizes the staff.

This swelling of staff interest led to an increased demand for data that could be analyzed and used for continued improvements. This in turn shifted the pressure back to quality management to collect, organize, and present data that could be used to test the rapidly growing hypotheses of workgroups and pilot units. Overall, this represented a healthy growth process for the development of quality and safety measures between QM and clinical staff.

Moving From a Top-Down Model to Hub and Spokes Model

Another key decision was to begin to move from a consultative-based model to lean transformation for attaining DOJ compliance. Under the consultative approach, staff were encouraged to find solutions through more traditional means centering around literature searches that would be used as guidelines. In practice, this caused a good deal of frustration and ultimately a mood of resigned passiveness among many clinical leaders who felt they were being force-fed predetermined solutions. With lean, the literature was considered but there was more of an emphasis on creatively tailoring unique solutions to our particular problems. The QM and Information Technology workgroups, facilitated by Breakthrough staff and utilizing A-3 thinking, were charged with devising strategies for compliance with the DOJ settlement agreement. Whereas other workgroups, such as the earlier described assessment workgroup, worked on specific areas of the settlement agreement, the QM and IT workgroups had to come up with the overall process for ensuring all details of the agreement were being addressed and that technology was available to ease data collection, analysis, and reporting.

The management product that resulted from the workgroups turned out to be a modified lean approach, because the volume of required performance indicators did not lend itself to the limited timeframe for completion. At this early point in our lean journey, we didn't have enough experience with lean to understand how it could be applied to all aspects of planning and management. The settlement agreement called for site visits to KCHC every 6 months by a team of subject matter experts; it was impossible to attempt to meet all established thresholds for success in such short periods of time. Therefore, the groups ended up selecting key components of compliance and applying the lean principles to each of these more limited areas. This was somewhat frustrating to the lean facilitators because the exercise was not a pure use of these principles. However, it was an opportunity to begin to educate a greater number of staff about the potential of lean.

Ultimately, the concept of equal workgroups gave way to a hub and spoke organizational model that put QM, Training, and Information Management in the center of the workgroups (see Figure 3.4).

This restructuring underscored the fact that data was the key ingredient for achieving the target states of all the workgroups. Of course, there was a two-way relationship in this model. It was expected that the workgroup would be able to define the parameters of needed data and QM would be able to produce it for them. This proved to be a chasm not easily overcome and a source of conflict within the organization because finding a happy medium between abstract hypotheses and concrete data poses many obstacles.

The first obstacle was attempting to define what information could reasonably be known. When dealing with quality and safety concerns, there are a vast number of factors that could conceivably impact on outcomes. For example, the workgroups would review a series of adverse outcomes and analyze what might have been done otherwise to avoid the unwanted result. Often the finding revolved around questionable clinical judgment on the part of the provider. But trying to narrow their findings down to a common denominator, such as the type of judgment error, proved an elusive goal.

Sometimes the workgroup would want QM to conduct chart reviews. However, it was not practical to devote the number of hours needed for such reviews or even to be able to quantify the results. Eventually, this led to a stratified chart review system. Supervisors would perform the highest level review and give feedback on overall clinical judgment. It was planned that clinical, discipline-specific peers (social work, MD, etc.) would give feedback similar to the supervisor's review; however, this part of the process never really took hold. Perhaps it was competing priorities, but more likely it was related to staff reluctance to participate in a peer review process. Although never explicitly stated, staff alluded to the potential inequities they perceived might occur if subjected to peer review: bias, competition, and personal agendas. As the culture changed, peer reviews gained acceptance and are now routinely done. The elements of quality and safety reserved for the chart reviewers were those associated with the comprehensiveness of an assessment or treatment plan. In particular, there was an emphasis to ensure that all potential "problems" identified in the range of completed assessments

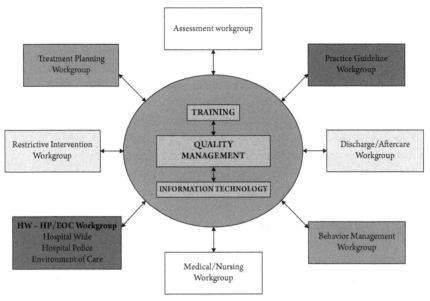

Figure 3.4 Workgroups.

had all required follow-up assessments and/or appropriate inclusion in the treatment plan.

Another problem we encountered was how to effectively tie this into meaningful staff training. It is one thing to have a supervisor complete a chart review and give critical feedback. That is a norm that is widely (even if sometimes begrudgingly) accepted in the health care industry. It is another thing to have the findings of a chart reviewer lead to some special training. The provider was less likely to accept any criticism and more likely to be resentful about being singled out for further education. It was the general approach to keep it "soft and gentle" depending on the circumstances. Preferably, the training might come on a one-to-one basis on the units and be presented in a collegial style. However, sometimes because of the pressurized setting, the training came down more like a hammer. Now sometimes a hammer is an appropriate and effective last resort, but the threat of the hammer sometimes cast the chart reviewers as the "bad guys." This has lessened over time, but we had to remain sensitive to how staff will react to differing levels of critical feedback.

Staff Development

It was not until early 2012 that BHS devoted specific time and energy to the creation of a staff development program. A 2-day retreat was held in which the beginnings of a program began to unfold through intense discussions. It became apparent that to achieve the goal of quality inpatient care, the need to support staff with their learning and training needs must be met.

Competency-based training and education is an integral component in developing and assessing individual performance. All employees need the opportunity to develop new skills and competencies and to become more connected with their customers.[8] Staff development now consists of five individual components: initial orientation, annual mandatory reviews, continuing education, discipline-specific training, and policy and procedure updates. These components serve to support and mentor staff. An environment of continued learning possibilities is intended to help staff develop and maintain the knowledge, skills, and abilities required to competently perform job duties, promote patient safety, and fully contribute to the achievement of our mission. A steering committee of key stakeholders was developed to administer the program of competency-based training and education.

Following the inception of the staff development program, we decided to have Staff Development reside within the Quality Department. In this manner, a clear linkage with education and performance improvement could occur. The action plans and data generated from the various quality activities were perceived to be a natural source of information and could serve to inform the educational needs assessment.

Electronic Chart Audit Tool

We were fortunate to be supported by a high level of technological support. This support emanated from the highest corporate levels and was carried out with enthusiasm by the Information Technology Department.

To start, BHS had the distinct advantage of having an excellent associate director for data management. This individual was a programmer by training but had extensive experience as a project director specializing in finding IT solutions for clinical performance improvement initiatives.

As is usually the case in such projects, the first step is to sit down with the clinical staff and solicit their input about the design and scope of the system. It is also usually the case that clinicians have difficulties in attempting to conceptualize how to isolate and frame data to produce meaningful reports. This is why an experienced project director is invaluable to drive the process. The range of effort given to the new quality reporting process varied greatly among clinical leadership. Some discipline heads were eager to embrace the technology and quickly generated meaningful reporting criteria. Others did not put in as much effort but were prodded along by suggestions from QM. An ongoing challenge was that the electronic health record was not based on current technology and therefore was not really effective for producing timely, user-friendly reports. There needed to be an electronic chart audit tool to make audit results instantly available to clinical leadership.

Our work resulted in the development of the Electronic Chart Audit Tool (ECAT). ECAT was devised as an electronic checklist where performance measures were preloaded into the system and chart reviewers would answer each question as either YES, NO, or NOT APPLICABLE. In addition, during data entry the name of the staff member responsible for the task could be selected from a pick-list. This enabled the system to assign an accountable person to each performance measure. Beyond the personal accountability of staff, ECAT enabled the organization to bolster its overall data integrity. In the past, it had been far too easy to collect reams of data by hand and then transcribe the findings to a spreadsheet without knowing who had collected the data and how it was collected. This method left the door open for transcription error and potential manipulation of data. However, ECAT made all this information instantly transparent. Essentially, it served as data source produced in the form of a visual management tool, which is so vital to lean implementation.

More than 30 separate audit tools were created, incorporating more than 500 performance measures that reflected the range DOJ and other regulatory requirements imposed on Behavioral Health. If performance was met for a certain measure, then it was calculated as part of the overall compliance. If performance was not met, then it was considered a "fallout" and factored against the compliance rate.

Beyond this, each performance measure was assigned to one of five categories: Assessment, Treatment Planning, Other Medical Record Documentation, Process, and Data Entry Error. This allowed for cross-reference across the tools as needed.

The highlight for clinical leadership was that the results of the chart audits were immediately published by ECAT into table and graphic forms upon submission of the completed tool by the chart reviewer. At a glance, the viewer was able to see compliance levels per indicator, per category, and per clinician. It also listed the finding by the name of the chart reviewer who entered the finding into the system. This closed the loop on accountability because it identified who was supposed to perform the neglected task and who made the determination that it was not done. Needless to say, this soon gained the attention of the clinicians who showed high numbers of fallouts. Although lean had helped us appreciate the need for data to understand and solve problems, it took us time to create the capacity for retrieving, analyzing, sharing, and reacting to data effectively.

Most of the early responses by clinicians with identified fallouts centered on attempts to sidestep the responsibility. Often, QM would receive irate communications indicating that the patient or task had been misidentified and the person had done everything expected of them. Unfortunately, this sometimes devolved into a contentious and nonproductive back-and-forth dialogue that fostered resentment and mistrust. Again, it is highly likely that the pressures associated with DOJ compliance accounted for some measure of the defensiveness on both sides. Most commonly, there would be a difference in interpretation about how to score certain performance measures. For example, a provider might have documented a disposition in a progress note rather than the section in the electronic health record designated for dispositions. If the chart reviewer had come upon the note, then credit might have been given for completion of the task. Some chart reviewers might interpret the measure rigidly and only look in the designated section. Others were more liberal and gave credit upon finding the progress note. This inconsistency in both documenting and scoring made it difficult to pinpoint the exact problems that needed improvement. The lean emphasis on standard of work, which would have helped reduce this variation and the re-work that resulted, was challenging due to constant changes being made to core processes.

Working through data discrepancies proved to be a fertile learning ground for clinicians and QM staff alike. The first response was to put the two accountable parties into a room and hash out the problem. The chart reviewer would explain what was being looked for in the chart, and the clinician would explain what they had done and why they had done it and where it could be found in the documentation. This led to the development of a "data dictionary" that explicitly listed the data elements being measured and the expected location of that data within the medical record. For example, the physician may have documented a patient's past illnesses in a progress note rather than the history and physical module. Although the information was in the record, it was not in a place where other team members would expect to find it. The presence of this dictionary helped reinforce the standard work and clarify any vagueness about data.

The outcomes of the clinician/chart reviewer disagreements varied from case to case. Sometimes clinicians were not aware of a particular policy and had in fact been noncompliant with the expected performance measure. Other times, the chart reviewer may have misapplied a policy or not looked in the proper location of the electronic health record. Either way, we learned to constantly update the "data dictionary" to assist all parties in completing and scoring documentation requirements and the need to following standard work gained traction.

However, no matter which side was right upon initial review, an effective educational process had been established to improve quality and safety. A new team relationship was fostered between clinical and quality staff. Just as important, if not more so, there was now an opportunity to recognize staff for performance that met or exceeded expectations. The same reviews that produced fallouts were also capable of identifying those clinicians who always, or nearly always, performed the task in the identified manner. This was useful to know because these individuals were exhibiting the type of "master clinician" attributes that were developed throughout Behavioral Health.

The ECAT reports were also highly versatile. Not only did ECAT instantly produce sharp looking graphics and tables, it was designed so that all data was readily exportable in an Excel format. This allowed for more sophisticated analysis of data across all audit tools.

The QM and Breakthrough staff immediately recognized the importance of this technological advancement. Now RIEs could be better planned through improved data sources and better monitored for sustainability in the future.

Dashboards

The clinical leadership embraced ECAT and quickly used it for training and competency purposes. The IT Department and BHS Data Center were operating at full throttle now and the next generation of improved technology came about in only a few short months. That improvement was the fully automated Behavioral Health Data Dashboard that displayed up-to-the-minute (literally) metrics directly downloaded from clinician's submissions into the electronic health record. It provided an automated chart review that did not require the manual chart audits done for ECAT.

Now, just because the technology came a short time after the introduction of ECAT, it does not mean that the feat was accomplished in that relatively short time frame. In fact, IT and QM had been working on the solution for about 2 years. Information Technology had to first create an internal database to collect the necessary information as it was entered into the electronic health record. This was a monumental task and the chief information officer and programming director were phenomenal in creating the application. It took painstaking review of thousands of potential data elements and creating a calculus for tracking the timeliness (such as in Table 3.1) and completion rates for a variety of assessments, treatment plans, and discharge planning documentation.

The database was designed to refresh every minute so that at any given time the viewer would have a 24-hour look back period to see length of stay, use of restraints, STAT medication orders, 1:1 close observation orders, and many other metrics that defined quality and safety measures. In addition, it had the capability to aggregate the collected data and instantly provide tables and graphs that displayed performance over any selected period of time.

If any single QM contribution had to be selected as the symbol of transformation, it would have to be the Data Dashboard (see Figure 3.5). The presence of accurate, live data coupled with a flexible aggregation feature completely changed how the organization could conduct business. This vision was now quite clear to QM, but it took a while for the magnitude of the accomplishment to be fully appreciated throughout the rest of BHS.

It took some convincing, but slowly the possibilities began to come to fruition. For example, a treatment team no longer needed to sit around for a half-hour of verbal reports to figure out how many patients were on restraints during the week. Nor did they have to check records and consult with one another about the number of STAT meds that were used the day before. All this information, whether in simple aggregate form or granular detail, was right at a touch of the fingertips. Now, the

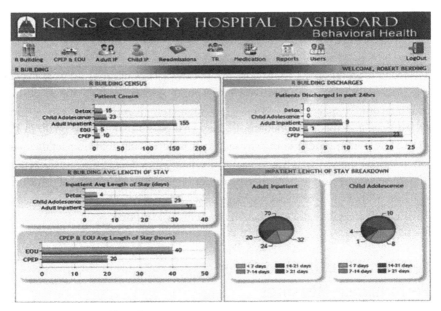

Figure 3.5 Data Dashboard.

organization was becoming more automated in producing lean visual management tools. No more waiting around for Breakthrough and QM staff to post graphic representations of projects. Rather, there was now a 24/7, real-time, at-a-glance picture available wherever there was a computer screen.

This opened a whole new world where data were not merely used for trend analysis, but now it could be used for daily unit management. The team leader could see at a glance how many patients were on one-to-one close observation and plan staffing patterns and patient clinical reviews for the day. In discussing a particular patient, the team could easily look at restraint usage or the use of 1:1s or stat IM medication over days or weeks and make decisions about behavioral interventions.

Another benefit is that the Data Dashboard inspired many staff to become inquisitive about trends in patient care. It is now an accepted routine that treatment team meetings take place around the computer screen. Staff can select different views and more fully consider patient care within the context of current outcomes. These views center around many of the RIEs, including Restraint Use and Length of Stay.

The Dashboard also empowered the staff to analyze data in new ways. Prior to the introduction of the Data Dashboard, staff had to wait for QM to publish data. If they wanted different timeframes or data elements, then they had to go back to QM and ask for the update. Although QM was always open to accommodating such requests, there were often times when it took several days to queue up and produce the report. Now staff merely need to select criteria and timeframe and the report is immediately on the screen and available for analysis.

Assuring Data Integrity

The quality assurance (QA) process requires us to produce accurate and complete automated data reports, a painstakingly laborious task. Countless hours are spent manually reconciling raw data with corresponding data fields in the electronic health record. To make matters worse, it is not merely an exercise that can be completed once and then forgotten about. Any change, no matter how small, in the record format may (and as known by sad experience, usually does) impact the manner in which information is transferred to the database and/or appears in the report. Thus, it was not uncommon after some minor system upgrade to receive panic calls that "the Data Dashboard isn't working right." It is essential to have a process for ongoing QA so as to maintain the integrity of the data reports.

Selecting Quality and Safety Performance Measures

Once the Data Dashboard was in place and the information validated as accurate and complete, it became much easier for staff to select and monitor performance measures. For example, the drill-down capability for use of restraints offered 32 elements of the event, including factors such as restraint type, duration, intervention attempts, and the provision of any safety measures. The real-time availability of this extensive data bank gave staff many options to monitor potential risk factors.

This newfound wealth of significant data, accessible to the BHS Steering Committee and any RIEs planned by that group, made understanding and prioritizing problems and improvement work much more manageable. This availability certainly made the reason for action, initial, and target states much clearer to all RIE participants. Further, the monitoring for "confirmed state" was usually already in place before the start of the RIE. Now that the monitoring capability had increased so dramatically, it was time for the reporting process to follow suit.

Quality Council—"Reporting Up"

The process for reporting the findings related to quality measures and projects was simultaneously evolving alongside the Breakthrough initiatives. In 2009, the BH reporting body known as the clinical council was changed to quality council. This group met on a monthly basis to discuss quality measures aside from the RIEs. The findings were presented by QM staff and often the local unit leadership would distance themselves from the outcomes by either dismissing the relevance of the data or refuting the accuracy of the findings. It was a dysfunctional, parallel universe.

In May 2011, a shift was implemented in the quality council that put the onus on the local unit leadership to explain any fallouts in qualitative measures and present corresponding corrective actions. The shift in responsibility caused staff to be anxious. Most were not accustomed to conceptualizing and implementing corrective action plans. However, a few trend setters began to emerge, most notably from the adult inpatient clinical leadership. These individuals took the charge seriously and spent long hours drilling down into the data.

Specialty subgroups began to emerge. More consideration was being given to the make-up of each sub-group assigned to analyze specific deficient performance measures. The members became more sophisticated in clearly discerning the issues, selecting the most pertinent data sets and measuring the outcomes. After a short while, the anxiousness turned to more positive types of energy. Teams were enthusiastic about being problem-solvers. Friendly competitions developed on a variety of quality and safety issues.

One significant change is that Breakthrough RIEs were now officially recognized as a viable performance improvement process. Despite having previously presented all the Breakthrough data to DOJ, Behavioral Health was criticized in hospital-wide reviews for a lack of department charted projects because the initiatives were not vetted through the former clinical council. This seemed odd to leaders throughout Behavioral Health because the number of RIEs was extremely high and the quality and safety improvements were palpable and a great source of pride for all Behavioral Health staff. We needed to communicate our evolving process better, and we recognized that the amount of data to be discussed at the quality council was simply too much to accomplish in a once-a-month format. So rather, the meetings were divided into multiple monthly meetings where each service would have sufficient time to present and discuss its performance improvement initiatives. We also made the BHS reporting formats more consistent with similar hospital-wide reports from other areas. In this way, the "reporting up" became much easier for other departments to understand the outcomes when presented at the main hospital Executive Quality Care Review Committee (EQCRC) and beyond.

Quality Rounds/Huddles—"Reporting Down"

Similarly to the evolution in Quality Council, the system for making quality rounds was progressing during this same period. In March 2009, administrative rounds were established as a means of sharing information throughout the units. For 1 hour, a large conference room would be filled with unit chiefs, assistant directors of nursing, head nurses, and other administrators. Each would give brief report on the prior day's occurrences and expected happenings for the upcoming day. The process was only useful for central leadership to become aware of unit-specific events and trends and was largely a poor use of time for treatment team members who might otherwise be interacting with their patients on the unit.

The emergence of the steering committee as the driving force behind BHS helped transform this process from waste to efficiency. One of the most important changes was the establishment of quality rounds as a replacement for the waste-laden administrative rounds.

Administrative rounds represented an early attempt to share information among clinical leaders. Rather, it became 2 hours of wasted time listening to reports of what had occurred 24 hours earlier. While the clinicians were packed in a conference room, the patients were becoming more and more frustrated by not being able to see a doctor.

In comparison, a Quality Rounds Team was headed by the clinical chief of service and included service and department directors. The rounds included six adult units, two adolescent units, one child unit, and the psychiatric emergency room. This concept was an extension of the gemba walk. Naturally, the group would inquire about lean standard work, but the discussions were not limited in that way. As such, it produced a "just do it" type of dialogue where problem solving was the priority.

A simple format was devised for this process. The Quality Rounds Team would visit two units per day on an alternating basis so that each unit was seen once a week. The treatment team would be notified the day before and the Quality Rounds Team would arrive at the conclusion of the regularly scheduled morning report. The iterative steps toward solidifying lean values within the organization led to a change in management style that valued data rather than avoiding it. This, in turn, fostered communication and helped tear down the defensive silo mentality that was prevalent among so many staff.

The expectation was that all units had monthly QM data posted on the bulletin boards for staff education purposes. The data reflected both Breakthrough and QM reports. Discussions would start from the level of staff awareness about the posted data and move toward suggestions for quality and safety improvements. The emphasis was to begin to have the line staff look at the data and offer some personal analysis about how conditions and outcomes might be improved on the units. Always, it was the Quality Rounds Team trying to gain a better understanding of what was happening on the unit while giving a strong voice to the treatment team members as change-makers.

Again, the reception varied from unit to unit. Some treatment teams appreciated and embraced an opportunity to be heard. Others were suspicious of the process and spoke only with prodding by the team members.

Of course, some units were having more success than others and this contributed to the amount of staff participation. For example, if a unit was experiencing a high number of incidents, the feedback from staff would typically be defensive and guarded. On the other hand, if a unit had some success in reducing the number of restraints or one-to-one close observations on the unit, then they would be eager to share their thoughts on the success.

Over time, most staff came to appreciate the opportunity to share their perceptions and recommendations. Many went on to participate in RIEs that reinforced the importance of their contributions. In particular, there was real ownership at the local level whenever a staff member participated in an RIE. It became much more than quality data posted on a bulletin board. It was a testament to their participation and a symbol of contribution to improved quality and safety.

After a time, however, the effect of quality rounds began to diminish. This is in part because the novelty of exposure to clinical leadership had worn off and some staff members were feeling like any extra meetings were a burden. However, there also appeared to be an "ebb and flow" based on goal attainment. That is, once a shorter term objective had been attained, the accompanying sense of urgency was reduced among the staff. The process needed to be tweaked with a more informal, situation-specific format. It was believed that the formal meeting might be replaced by a more informal "huddle" where staff could discuss emerging issues in a succinct manner.

A quality huddle concept was launched to freshen up the process. The focus was on any performance measure that was not making some anticipated rate of improvement. Rather than going up to individual units, department heads and/or specific unit staff would be invited to attend a brainstorming session to arrive at solutions as problems were identified, without waiting for an event to be planned.

These huddles were supplemented by unit visits to observe the outcome of the huddle discussions. The idea was to put a plan together quickly and then go up to the units to test it out. The testing was akin to the rapid experiment phase of an RIE. An emphasis was also put on tying huddles to quality council meetings. Both RIEs and just do its would be discussed on the unit in anticipation of the formal report. This structure now more fully involved the whole staff in the performance improvement process. Ultimately, this real-time problem-solving approach proved more effective for engaging staff and "reporting down" through the units.

Regression and Reinvention

Organizations that boast a true culture committed to quality and safety have the uncanny ability to identify, measure, and evaluate those critical elements of performance that derive from the true north metrics. Efforts are centered around critical clinical processes, outcomes, financial and strategic business results, and the patient experience. Identifying a framework that yields the greatest return on investment of time, effort, and money while achieving services deemed excellent beyond compliance is an aim of both performance improvement and Breakthrough initiatives.

Behavioral Health Services accomplished a great deal in short order. The CPEP-ER had substantially improved in becoming a more efficient and safe environment. Patients routinely received comprehensive assessments in timely fashion, and the communications among staff included a greater level of detail that could be incorporated into the treatment planning process. Staff roles were better defined as a result of all the new work standards developed through RIEs. Reliable and accurate data was readily available through the Dashboard. The bright and clean environment of the "R" building was the icing on the cake.

Yet, as with all good things, there was still much work to be done. Despite some early successes in breaking down the "silo mentality" within the organization, it slowly began to creep back into the equation now as "silos of excellence." This probably occurred for a number of reasons. First, silos are facially appealing for validating the efforts and viewpoints of the individual disciplines. It is much more comfortable for physicians, nurses, social workers, and other health care professionals to use the language and approach of their training with each other to discuss patient outcomes. Likewise, staff assigned to particular services may easily fall into silo dialogues based on whether they work with adults, adolescents, or children.

Staff turnover is another erosion factor in attempting to sustain cohesive, transdisciplinary treatment teams. BHS is a large operation with a challenging patient population and, as such, has experienced a significant amount of turnover. These new staff members are more likely to seek intradisciplinary silos because it shrinks the universe of information that needs to be processed when completing assigned tasks.

Perhaps most importantly, silos tend to gain strength when needed for survival in the workplace. Behavioral Health is a stressful field to begin with, but when put under the spotlight of a federal government law enforcement branch, it can become downright threatening to professional reputation. Because of this elevated pressure, it was not uncommon for some BHS staff to feel under knee-jerk attack from its own leadership if there was any hint of noncompliance with the DOJ settlement agreement.

The takeaway here was that to tear down silos and not have them rise up again rapidly, there would need to be an ongoing commitment to organizational education and trust among all the players that accountability for missed thresholds would not fall unfairly upon a single person or group. This is a particularly challenging standard to maintain but leadership and staff have both made good-faith efforts to live by it.

Nurse managers and unit chiefs were selected as the focal point unit leaders. A series of educational sessions were developed and presented with the expectation that the information be carried back to the unit level. The initial session included an introduction to the Plan—Do—Check—Act (P—D—C—A) methodology as this was the methodology identified by the organization for performance improvement. In creating the curriculum for this educational offering, the Quality leadership

---

Lessons Learned

Teaching on the units can be much more efficient and sustainable than in the classroom. In late 2011, the concept of bringing quality back to the bedside was re-invented during one of the quality huddles. Staff participation and engagement in Breakthrough activities was thriving, yet the link between quality and day-to-day activities needed a reinvigorating shot in the arm. So, to connect the dots, the quality leadership went back to the gemba.

---

felt strongly about highlighting the fact that P—D—C—A is actually embedded in A3 thinking reinforcing the congruency between performance improvement and Breakthrough. This effort was well received by the units and is now a cornerstone of the quality and safety improvement process. Lean = improvement process.

Quality Council Expansion—Including Risk Management

Also in late 2011, it became evident to senior administrative leadership that enhanced clinical involvement was needed in both quality council and the Special Incident Review Committee (SIRC) —the two main forums for quality and safety. This senior team felt weighed down with owning the administrative processes for these meetings as well as carrying much of the load with respect to interpreting, analyzing, and responding to the data. Not that the team did not feel this to be their responsibility. Rather, it was out of the desire to ensure a thorough drill down—to the patient level, if necessary—to truly understand the story that the data represented and to come up with a plan of correction that was actionable at the unit level.

Utilizing A3 thinking, the team identified a target state in which staff members were actively involved in each step of the improvement cycle. Essentially, a tiered approach to quality and safety was adopted for use by the group. The functions and responsibilities of the committee remained constant, which included data analysis and sanctioning any associated corrective action plans.

However, two new groups emerged. The first was a core team, consisting of key discipline leaders. This group was charged with supporting the process owner for the quality council and SIRC and providing guidance to the second emerging group, the subcommittee. This arrangement mirrored that of the facilitators and sensei in the Breakthrough model. The core team would act as sensei, or teacher, while the subcommittee took on the role of facilitator, or person(s) who lead the action. The subcommittee turned out to be the critical new element, or missing link, which bridged the gap and filled the void between the conference room and the bedside. They now did the analysis at the local clinical level (unit, CPEP, etc.) and reported it to the quality council and SIRC, who could then focus on trends and higher level root causes and systems solutions.

The existing quality and safety monitoring practices remained intact—at least at the onset. Data was collected in a manner consistent with current practices. However, rather than first distributing data to the core group, it was initially reviewed and analyzed by the subcommittee. Unit leadership and line staff now had the opportunity to receive and digest data rather than simply having the information posted on a bulletin board. Communication was growing by leaps and bounds and it was only natural that a large scale quality and safety event should follow. By this point, the organization continued to do events on at least a monthly basis and had indoctrinated A3 thinking into all aspects of management.

Quality Fair

During a quality huddle, the chief of service asked those present if they thought that the department would be in a position to host a quality fair to showcase their efforts. The question was posed softly and with a look that implied she would take back the words if at all possible. Although no one openly came out in opposition, there was not much demonstrable enthusiasm for the idea. Truth be told, fear was probably the prevailing emotion at the time. The question eventually was re-framed into a statement of fact—BHS will showcase quality and safety by hosting its own internal fair. The fair would serve a dual purpose: (1) to share the knowledge gained in achieving successful outcomes, and (2) celebrate the contributions of the team members. The presentations were to be given by front-line staff who participated in the development and implementation of each project. Invitations were extended throughout the whole hospital.

BHS boasted an array of chartered performance improvement initiatives, many emanating from Breakthrough RIEs. It would have only natural that these projects would take center stage at the fair. However, the Chief of Service had another plan in mind. The directive was that each and every unit would be represented to showcase their work. As soon as the basic details such as location and times were identified, the wheels were set in motion.

The A3 model thinking was the platform by which each unit organized and assembled their performance improvement project. The groups demonstrated a basic comfort level with the terminology and practices despite having limited leadership experience in A3 completion. Nurse managers and unit chiefs labored over large sheets of paper populating the various A3 boxes.

The quality huddle participants were more experienced with A3 completion and met regularly with unit staff to assist their progress. Each box on the grid was discussed in detail to include all of the appropriate information. Slowly over time, things began to take shape. Unit staff made numerous calls to Q&C asking for various data elements but with a new sense of sophistication. The clinicians were telling the Data Shop which elements were necessary and how they wished them to be displayed. Relationships between actions taken and various elements of performance were explored in the hopes of finding meaningful correlation.

The Quality Fair day arrived and after setting one foot into the gymnasium where it was held, it was evident—BHS was an energized and unified department of engaged staff. The excitement and enthusiasm in the room were palpable. As one nurse stated, the fair "is giving me goose bumps!" Each and every unit was represented and proud to show off their work, Months later, the performance gains displayed at the fair were still being sustained at the increased level of improvement (see Figure 3.6).

One project, which was showcased at the far corner of the room, stood out from the others. Perhaps it was because the staff stood proudly by the display and were not willing to relinquish their spot. However, when your turn came to stand in front of their display, it was reminiscent of childhood science fair projects. As you listened to the story that was unfolding on the inpatient child and adolescent unit, it was apparent that something exceptional was on display.

Early on, the child and adolescent unit stood out as somewhat of a maverick group. When core quality council members showed up to participate in the quality subcommittee session, they expected to find a formal and structured meeting. Such was not the case. The medical director described that mechanism in which quality and safety data was reviewed and analyzed was by going to the gemba. Although he may not have used the word *gemba*, it was clearly articulated that the data was presented on the unit and discussed during morning report and unit rounds. This

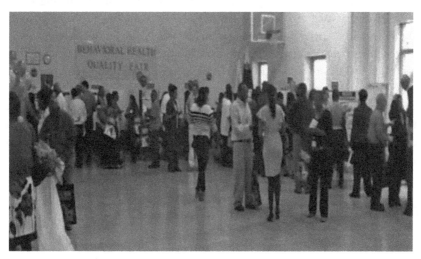

Figure 3.6 Quality fair.

informal approach allowed the process to become a living and breathing practice. So it came to no surprise that the unit's performance improvement project was unequivocally driven by the entire staff.

Their project was aimed at reducing high-risk behaviors in the child and adolescent inpatient unit while employing the least restrictive measures. This aim was in alignment with all of the strategic goals of the service. Their reason for action was that high-risk behaviors (assault, self-harm, suicide, or sexual acting out) imposes a significant threat for safety of patients and staff.

The team based their interventions on the belief that these behaviors could be reduced by instituting a system of early identification of high-risk groups, coupled with targeted pre-emptive plans that were responsive to the needs of the patient. Due diligence was applied when reviewing the data, including restraint rates, one-to-one observation usage, STAT medications, assaults, and fights. Measures of success were set and action plans rolled out for unit-wide implementation. These included the team's ability to identify early each day the patient most at risk and to allocate staffing resources around the patient as a preventative mechanism. Soon the "patient of the day" practice was yielding positive results. Visual displays were incorporated into the décor of the unit, including a white board identifying the number of restraint free days. Incident review was conducted both in real time and retrospectively to gather as much information as possible. Ongoing feedback to all staff was built into the plan to keep everyone abreast of the status and to implement course correction if need be. The effectiveness of this initiative was highlighted during a subsequent joint commission site survey when the "patient of the day" concept was identified as a unique best practice by the survey team.

The concept was a simple one. The patient of the day was the one who could most reasonably have been expected to be involved in an incident yet refrained from any untoward behavior. Such high-risk patients were rewarded for avoiding aggressive behavior that might have otherwise led to 1:1 observation, STAT medications, and/or restraints. Anecdotally, there appears to be a positive relationship between nonaggressive behavior and regularly scheduled "therapeutic check-ins" where patients know staff will meet with them at designated times throughout the day.

When the BHS Deputy Executive Director indicated at a TMT meeting that he would like to initiate a practice of acknowledging individuals or teams who have embodied the mission, vision, and goals of the service, there was an immediate consensus among the group. Clearly, the Child and Adolescent unit was the unanimous choice. It was truly fitting that the award was named to match the achievement—the Lotus Award.

Improved Quality and Safety Lead to Financial Gain

As yet, has BHS arrived at it goals? The answer is a resounding and emphatic NO. For, if BHS had "arrived," then it would mean an end to the journey. In reality the journey towards quality and safety has no end. The bar is always being raised, competition stiff, and demand high. The cycle of evolution remains an ongoing, constant trek. However, one thing is for certain, quality and safety are now true north metrics for BHS.

Over the prior few years, many substantial improvements were realized and staff felt a renewed sense of pride and accomplishment for the outcomes. The most obvious outcomes were easily observable; patients were now receiving services in a manner that was within generally accepted professional standards; some patients with long histories of violence were having more tranquil inpatient stays, and; so many staff felt and exuded a personal commitment to the results of an RIE in which they had been a personal participant.

Looking back to the starting point, BHS is a significantly safer place than it was prior to DOJ and plaintiff investigations. Although the scope of reporting assaults has been widened so as to be overly-inclusive of all aggressive occurrences, the serious assault rate has trended down over time. It is also relevant that the number of incidents with serious injuries has gone down significantly as well. The feeling of safety can be elusive in an environment where many of the residents are involuntarily committed for dangerous behavior. Yet on more days than others, the majority of units operate quietly and without incident. It has certainly come a long way from the days of the uncontrollable barrages and survivalist barricades in "G" Building.

It is even more gratifying that quality has bloomed, like the lotus that is our symbol, from a nearly nonexistent beginning to a center of excellence. Professionals from around the world have come to observe the strides in the provision of quality programs and services. Quality now has form. There are benchmarks for everything from initial diagnosis to recidivism. Beyond that, the unit staff has been empowered to analyze the data and make decisions that propel quality on a daily basis.

But for those on the financial side of the equation, the improvements also began to register on the ledger sheet; reduced 1:1 meant less need for agency staff and overtime; decreased LOS translated into an improved percentage of reimbursable days; and improved outpatient workflows led to more revenue. The pioneering of the true north metrics of quality and safety had led the inevitable linkage of their true north counterpart, improved profitability.

Notes

1. Bicheno J., Holweg M. (2009). *The Lean Toolbox: The Essential Guide to Lean Transformation*, fourth edition (pp. 4–17). Buckingham, England: PICSIE Books.
2. Arthur, J. (2011). *Lean Six Sigma Demystified*, second edition (pp. 47–48). New York: McGraw-Hill.
3. Miller L.M. (2011). *Lean Culture: The Leader's Guide* (p. 13). Annapolis, MD: LM Miller Publisher.

4. Leape L. (1994). Error in medicine. *Journal of the American Medical Association*, 272(23): 1851–1857.
5. Agency for Healthcare Research and Quality. TeamSTEPPS Pocket Guide Version 06.1, June 2010.
6. Jackson T.L., Ed. (2009). *5S for Healthcare* (p. 27). Boca Raton, FL: CRC Press, Taylor and Francis Group.
7. Liker J.K. (2004). *The Toyata Way: 14 Management Principles for the World's Greatest Manufacturer* (p. 223). New York: McGraw-Hill.
8. Price M., Mores W., Elliotte H.M. (2011). *Building High Performance Government Through Lean Six Sigma* (p. 13). New York: McGraw-Hill.

4

Financial Benefits of Lean

MARLENE ZURACK, ROSLYN S. WEINSTEIN, AND GEORGE PROCTOR

When we first began our lean effort at the enterprise level at the Health and Hospitals Corporation (HHC), we were guided by our sensei to identify our "burning platform." This statement was intended to be the defining problem that our lean work was designed to address and the opening salvo to our first enterprise transformational plan of care (TPOC), a lean agenda set by organizational leaders. However, at that time, the end of 2007, our financial situation had never been better. We had just negotiated a deal with New York City and New York State that brought in new revenue, and we had unprecedented support from Mayor Michael R. Bloomberg as evidenced by a $1.2 billion city-financed major modernization program in which half of our facilities were rebuilt. Reflecting the newness of lean for us—our "waste goggles" were not yet developed—our platform could probably be more accurately described as smoldering rather than burning; it read like our mission statement tailored to instill a general desire to improve.

Our organization is built on a history measured in centuries; many of our hospitals have celebrated anniversaries in excess of 150 years. With its proud legacy of providing quality health care to everyone regardless of ability to pay, HHC is very much interwoven into the fabric of New York City.

From the top down we are a leadership team consisting of corporate senior vice presidents aligned to functional areas—the classic "C" suite, chief financial officer, chief medical officer, chief operating officer—with enterprise-wide responsibilities. Each operational network, representing several major health care facilities in New York City, is led by a network senior vice president. Although we all work for the same president and the same board, we are not immune from a classic "us-against-them" mindset: the bureaucrats downtown versus the real people doing the real work at the facilities or, from the other perspective, the caretakers versus the doers.

From the bottom up we employ more than 40,000 health care professionals and serve 1.3 million patients. Our revenues approach $7 billion a year. The scope and complexity of this organization is breathtaking; from the inside, one can feel like

Alice in Wonderland. Making change uniformly or even consistently or even in the same direction is a heroic effort. Accordingly, developing a model for managing daily improvement and measuring return on investment using lean at HHC was a very serious and risky undertaking.

In this chapter we will share our experiences in transforming HHC using lean principles in finance and revenue cycle processes, and our attempt to spread the practice of measuring and aligning improvement, including return on investment. HHC is only approaching the end of Act I of this play and will likely see many twists and turns before we conclude Act III. We aspire, at some point, to be a truly lean organization. This chapter will also cover the specific lean experience of the Corporate Finance Division, beginning at the onset of HHC's lean journey and continuing until the present. We will start with an overview of HHC's finances. Next will be a review of the Corporate Finance Division's lean journey. We will also present the experiences of two hospitals very much engaged in applying lean to finance issues, Woodhull Medical and Mental Health Center and Kings County Hospital Center. These experiences will shed light on the difficulties and importance of embedding the concept of return on investment into the organizational culture while trying to align with corporate strategic priorities.

Fundamentals of Health and Hospitals Corporation's Finances Before Lean

In the fall of 2007, HHC had an A credit rating from Moody's, Standard and Poor's, and Fitch. To understand the dichotomy of a public hospital system with a troubled financial and management past and a credit rating better than many private hospital systems, one needs to understand the fundamentals of HHC finance.

The corporation's financial condition is defined in part by the circumstances of its creation and its current relationship with New York City. As a large urban center drawing its population from multiple historic waves of immigration from various parts of the world, New York City developed a large number of public hospitals throughout the five boroughs, many of which were originally built to address the polio and tuberculosis epidemics. The New York City budget for fiscal years 1968 to 1969 included funding for 27 hospitals with a total bed capacity of 18,356 and a budget of $416 million, representing 7% of the city budget.

HHC was created from the New York City Department of Hospitals in 1969 as an independent public benefit corporation; its creation was cemented in state law and through an operating agreement and a lease of real property signed by Mayor John Lindsay and HHC's first president, Joseph English. The thinking was that the corporation would be better able than the city to take advantage of two new programs created contemporaneously by the federal government as part of the "Great Society," Medicaid and Medicare.

The creation of Medicaid was an opportunity for the city to offset some of the costs it bore for its large public hospital and public health systems but came with the requirement that the city itself contribute 25% of the costs to the program, the state commit another 25%, and the remaining 50% was the federal share. In many ways, the city's move to dissociate from its public hospitals began a tug of war on several fronts. First, it put the city in the position of forcing the corporation's management to become more efficient. Second, it encouraged the corporation to seek funding from the state and federal governments through Medicaid and Medicare. The advent of Medicaid and Medicare made government a very large investor in health insurance.

The state law creating the corporation established some ground rules for the future relationship with the city and anticipated that details would be worked out as part of an operating agreement. The terms of the relationship established by the Operating Agreement, dated June 16, 1970, noted that the corporation is responsible for the control, maintenance, and provision of health services to the residents of the city regardless of ability to pay and included a provision whereby the city leased facilities to the corporation for an annual rental of one dollar for a term coexistent with the life of the corporation. The Operating Agreement also provides that the city shall bargain for and approve labor agreements on behalf of the corporation, and the city shall indemnify the corporation and its affiliates for liabilities incurred in connection with the delivery of health services, including administrative acts and malpractice claims.

The state law requires the city to provide an annual minimum of $175 million to the corporation for the provision of health care services. This minimum subsidy must be adjusted annually to reflect inflation, changes in reimbursement rates, and increases in services rendered for which no compensation from third-party sources is available. In computing its minimum subsidy to meet this requirement, the city has included its share of Medicaid payments to the corporation.

From 1970 through 1992, the city maintained a watchful eye on HHC's expense budget, analyzing and approving line item budgets. However, in 1992 the city and HHC recast their relationship. HHC was given much greater autonomy in its operations and the city stopped providing substantial direct subsidy. In 1973, 60% of HHC's budget came from direct city support. By 1992, less than 8% of HHC's budget came from direct city support.

Two things happened in the early 1990s that changed HHC's relationship with the city dramatically. The city negotiated with the state and the federal government to access disproportionate share hospital (DSH) and upper payment limit (UPL) matching funds to support the corporation's operations. As a result, an increasing percentage of the corporation's city-funded operating revenue has come from Medicaid and Supplemental Medicaid rather than from direct general city support. DSH is a federal program that was created to provide federal Medicaid payments to hospitals to cover their unreimbursed costs for treating a disproportionate share of

Medicaid and uninsured patients. UPL is a regulation in the federal Medicaid program that allows states to pay hospital inpatient and outpatient rates that approximate what would have been paid under Medicare. The federal government funds half of the DSH and UPL payments to the corporation, and the city bears the full nonfederal share for the other half of these payments. A state statute authorizes that these payments be made by the city; the state submits the requisite federal requests for approval but does not participate financially.

In addition, the corporation exercised its authority to issue revenue bonds to support its capital programs. The city has shown great support for HHC by financing the recent capital program. Prior to 1992, all of HHC's capital improvements were funded with New York City debt.

More than one-third of HHC's 1.3 million patients are uninsured; another two-thirds are insured through a combination of Medicaid, Medicaid-managed care, Medicare, and commercial insurance; and HHC receives payments from the city for care of the city's prisoners and uniformed service workers. Given this payer mix, it is no wonder that HHC depends on support from New York City. In recent years, the city demonstrated continued support for HHC by significantly increasing its contribution to Supplemental Medicaid payments received by the corporation. Unfortunately, sustaining Supplemental Medicaid revenues is a complex battle with three levels of government—city, state, and federal. Each level requires the corporation to demonstrate that it is working as best it can to improve quality and service levels at reduced costs.

In 2008, the economic crisis led to a $1.2 billion budget gap for HHC. A state budget crisis and a reformed state payment methodology resulted in $500 million in cuts to HHC's Medicaid collections. Losses in the New York City pension fund investment returns required a $400 million increase to HHC's employer contributions. City budget cuts reduced revenue, interest earnings declined, and the number of uninsured patients steadily grew. To close this gap, HHC initiated a cost containment plan in 2009 and a restructuring program in 2010, each worth about $300 million. In addition, the city added matching funds and the state authorized increases to federal Supplemental Medicaid payments.

In late 2008, about 1 year into Breakthrough (the name HHC has given its lean efforts), it was time for leadership to update the enterprise-level transformational plan of care (ETPOC) to reflect this new and stark reality. The corporation projected that without dramatic transformation, we would see a $1.2 billion gap in our $7 billion budget within 2 fiscal years. As the economy rapidly declined, government budgets were stressed. Deep cuts in Medicaid and city funds along with steep increases in pension and health insurance expense brought us to this unhappy fate. Not surprisingly, when we met to update our ETPOC this time, we were all engaged around the need to use lean to save $100 million in the next fiscal year. How these things called value stream and rapid improvement events would produce this was less clear, but not too many platforms burn hotter than this. At this early juncture the corporate CFO, who has a background in process improvement strategies, became one of the most senior leaders in the corporation to entrust the achievement of major corporate priorities to lean solutions. The value of the CFO's early adoption has benefited the corporation through continuously challenging times, both through her adoption of lean tools and philosophy in specific areas of revenue cycle and finance and through her willingness to deeply embed lean thinking throughout the daily operation of her division. In 2010, the federal Affordable Care Act was passed, challenging HHC to form new partnerships with other providers, to significantly upgrade its electronic medical record system and to aggressively pursue a model of care that enhances preventive and primary care. At the same time, New York State began a major redesign of its Medicaid program. Taken together, these challenges have kept the management of HHC on a multiyear rollercoaster.

Corporate Finance's Use of Lean to Manage Through Extreme Change

In many ways the early adoption of lean by the Finance Department was fortunate. The department was able to cut its teeth on some initial value streams before the pressure to produce results intensified. At first we focused on improving the accuracy of our reporting, creating standard work for key cost report schedules and for insuring data accuracy. These early events took in the "voice of the customer," in this case defined as our facilities, and provided the opportunity to practice using standard work and a structured process for monitoring the maintenance of changes. We next used lean to prepare standard workflows to support the implementation of a new Revenue Cycle Management System. This first wave of effort produced about $4 million in savings by reducing duplicate employee health insurance, reducing payments to the city for the cost of Medicare for employees, and simplifying administrative processes.

We experimented with different tools, team composition, and venues, and consequently our value streams often lost focus. We tended to overscope our events and not to do enough preparatory work before the improvement events, and we failed to complete all of our postevent activities and ignored sustainment altogether. We attempted to create a profit and loss report by facility by service line but failed to roll it out across the corporation. In fact, we have added this back to our plan for next year.

As part of the 2009 restructuring program, corporate finance agreed to generate $100 million a year in additional revenue—one-third of the corporation's total program target of $300 million in revenue enhancements and expenditure cuts. Finance would open an enterprise-wide "Charge Capture" value stream. We were in such a rush we held three simultaneous value stream analysis events: (1) system improvements; (2) inpatient and long-term care charge capture, and (3) outpatient charge capture. The scope seemed broader than the seven seas.

Several key members of the senior staff at corporate finance became process owners of multiple simultaneous corporate-wide improvements. What were we thinking? We spent a lot of time creating standard work, much of which was never implemented. We learned a lot about lean but a lot of the learning came from our mistakes and some staff felt overburdened by the challenge.

One wonderful thing happened in two areas. We used lean on projects that we had tried to implement, over a significant period of time, with more traditional project management methods. When we used lean to develop workflows for our new Revenue Cycle Management Information Technology System, we were able to move and manage the project, delivering all of our documents to our vendor on time and engaging the organization deeply. Also, we dusted off our Documentation and Coding Improvement Initiative and implemented it broadly and deeply throughout the corporation. These two projects alone generated $86 million in additional revenue.

These two projects alone generated $86 million in additional revenue. The following Figure shows the growth in financial benefits accruing from lean activity over time. In just under 6 years, our cumulative cost savings and new revenue reached $347 million (see Figure 4.1).

We celebrated our successes and learned from our mistakes but still did not embed lean into our daily life. In 2011, the start of corporate finance's fourth year with lean, we decided to embed it into our daily life. This required our senior team to learn to be facilitators—including the corporate CFO. We now have three embedded facilitators and three others in training within the division. All of our facilitators

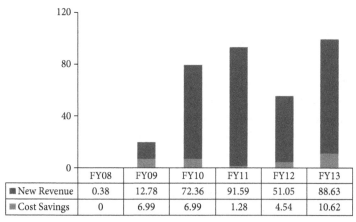

	FY08	FY09	FY10	FY11	FY12	FY13
■ New Revenue	0.38	12.78	72.36	91.59	51.05	88.63
■ Cost Savings	0	6.99	6.99	1.28	4.54	10.62

Source: NYCHHC Enterprise Breakthrough Office

Figure 4.1 Financial Benefit from Lean Activity—Enterprise-Wide, All Activities.
Numbers in millions. Includes new revenue and cost savings associated with one-time and ongoing Breakthrough activity. Source: Enterprise Steering Committee Monthly Report, June 2013, NYCHHC.

and process owners get regular training from our external sensei and we do not start a value stream without conducting substantive prework, establishing metrics, and setting up a governance structure. Eighty-five percent of staff in corporate finance has participated in at least one lean event. And we have all adopted A3 thinking into our routines. This year we are hoping to achieve another $20 million in additional revenue from enterprise revenue cycle improvements alone.

From the beginning of our lean work, we struggled to capture return on investment at all levels—rapid improvement events (RIEs), value stream, site, and enterprise. In hindsight, we probably expected both too much from the individual RIEs and too little from the value stream level. We expected that each RIE should influence all five of our true north dimensions, including quality/safety, human development, finance, throughput, and growth, with each RIE. We were disappointed when a standard work event reduced variation and decreased processing time but savings or new revenue opportunity was impossible to capture. It took us time to learn that only when sufficient improvements had taken place—when enough of the rocks in the road had been removed—could value flow. It takes a lot of steps to provide a service, collect adequate documentation, submit a bill, deal with denials, and finally receive some portion of the cost of the service back in revenue. As we tried to scope RIEs to be narrow and deep versus wide and shallow, it would be a rare RIE that could solve enough of these processes to achieve the end result of revenue or even, in our low-margin world, significant savings. Eventually we learned to expect driver metrics—flow, handoffs, variation, steps, physical space, changes in processes—to move as a result of RIEs and for metrics that required long sequences of solutions to be joined effectively on a consistent and repeated basis—revenue and savings, clinical outcomes, length of stay—to see movement at the value stream or even the site level.

It should be said that during prior RIEs, we had occasionally come up with either revenue or cost savings from single events, and in fact, some of these were significant. But these gains were exceptions and could not be produced with the reliability required to achieve the type of stretch targets we needed. Whether we were looking for financial benefit from RIEs or at the aggregate, value stream level, we realized that an even more fundamental problem we had was a lack of confidence and a process for monetizing improvements. Across sites, variations in definitions (regarding who was responsible for setting targets, collecting information, and verifying results) led to paralysis and a lack of credibility in anything that was produced. Finally, after several years struggling with this issue, we had enough experience to pull together a group of site CFOs, the corporate CFO, and a few process owners to investigate the problem and develop a solution.

Getting to this point we learned a few things. First, we went to a trusted sister organization, Denver Health, and asked them to tell us again what they had told us a couple of years earlier but that, at that time, we were too early in our journey to understand. Denver Health, the public health and hospital system in Colorado, shared their experience from key finance, lean, and clinical perspectives. They helped us understand what types of improvements could be expected to produce results and how conservative measurement leant credibility to the numbers, and they described their structure for benefit accountability. As a result, we developed standard work for monetizing results that included who set targets, the role of the CFO in verifying results and owning the data, and most importantly for sites, detailed cost and revenue analysis steps for the most frequent financial benefits accrued in the five largest value streams.

Woodhull's Experience With Return on Investment

Woodhull Medical and Mental Health Center contributed significantly to the development of standard work for monetizing lean benefits. The Woodhull CFO spent months analyzing cost and revenue at the service and cost center level, looking at direct and indirect personnel costs and supply costs and tracing the complex constellation of revenue that is unique to our hospital system. With the large percentage of uninsured and self-pay patients seen at HHC facilities, as well as the distributions from various state and federal pools described earlier in this chapter, coming up with a net revenue or savings number was not easy and would need thoroughly documented and verifiable calculations to pass muster. Woodhull's work resulted in an ROI template that identifies the benefits and savings of a RIE, including the cost of staff time in the event, any consultant and subject matter expert costs, and even the cost of meals provided for team members. The template, which is available to all sites, also contains the narrative for RIE sustainment associated with the Completion Plan from each event. Ultimately, through a consensus process with all CFOs, the corporate CFO signed off on a somewhat less complex process for enterprise roll-up of financial benefits. We realized that differences between sites— especially in rates and historically based cost structures—required that we simplify the process for comparability. Standardizing how we defined and captured financial benefits from lean resulted in more frequent and consistent reporting by sites. This standard work is included below as Boxes 4.1A and 4.1B.

Kings County Hospital Center Behavioral Health Experience

Over the last several years many have described the importance of ambulatory care as the foundation for curbing costs within the health care market. However, the hospital-based outpatient department has not operated at peak efficiency so the theory has never been proven. As inpatient psychiatric reimbursement formulas suffer yearly cuts, the role of the outpatient department (OPD) has become evident. In

Box 4.1A Standard Work for Financial Contributions

Roles, Validation, and Reporting

Workflow	CFO designated as resource to site EST	Financial SME designated for VSSTs	Potential financial target identified for value stream	Potential financial targets identified for RIEs	Achievement reviewed by SME 30/60/90 days post-event	CFO validates achievement/benefit	Benefit reviewed by ESC	Benefits reported to Enterprise SC	Process Step
									Process Trigger

Work Sequence

1. Facility CFO is a resource to the site steering team.

2. CFO or designee is member of the facility executive steering team (EST). The CFO/designee(s) will assist the EST in establishing financial measures and targets for the TPOC and value streams, as well as in interpreting and reporting financial achievements/contributions resulting from Breakthrough activity.

3. The CFO will designate an appropriate individual to:
   - either be a member of each Value Stream Steering Team (VSST) or serve as a financial subject matter| expert (SME) for each value stream; and
   - provide consultation for the development of financial measures and targets for each RIE that has the potential for monetization.

4. During the RIE prework phase, the financial SME will provide guidance to the Process Owner, Facilitator, and Team Leader to identify potential opportunities to achieve financial benefits from the RIE, to establish associated measures and targets, and to identify the data collection method and time anticipated time frame for achievement of these targets. The Monetization Standard Work will be used to guide the selection and definition of measures.

5. The projected financial benefit shall be included in the RIE Confirmed State.

6. Progress toward RIE financial achievement will be monitored and reported by the financial SME to:
   - the CFO for verification; and,
   - after verification, the BDO or BDO designee for inclusion by the BDO in 30/60/90 post-event reports to the event PO and VSST at appropriate intervals.

7. The facility CFO ensures the reporting of financial contributions from each "monetized" event to the Enterprise Breakthrough Office for inclusion in monthly reports to the ESC by the 10th of each month following the reporting month.
   - The Monetization Standard Work will be used to guide the validation of financial contributions.
   - The Financial Contribution Reporting Form will be used to report all financial information to the Enterprise Breakthrough Office.

8. The Enterprise Breakthrough Office will include all facilities' financial contributions in the monthly report to the Enterprise Steering Committee.

Box 4.1B Standard Work for Financial Contributions

Development and Reporting of Countermeasures Site Financial Steering Team

Workflow	Box 8 is not achieved	PO conducts gap analysis	PO develops CM	VSST Reviews CM	VSST may make recommendations to PO and site EST	Makes recommendations as needed to VSST PO & CFO	If CMs, so noted in report to ESC	PO monitors ongoing contributions	Process Step / Process Trigger

Work Sequence

1. Process Owner identifies that financial contribution goal(s) are not being achieved.

2. Process Owner analyzes cause for underachievement and develops countermeasure to address root cause. Countermeasure may range from simple steps to resolving a small defect in the process (JDI), to initiating an RIE to analyze the problem and develop a new solution approach.

3. Process Owner submits the countermeasure to the Value Stream Steering Team (VSST) for review.

4. VSST reviews countermeasure and may make recommendations to the Process Owner and the facility Executive Steering Team.

5. Facility Executive Steering Team reviews all countermeasures and makes recommendations for follow-up as needed to the Process Owner, CFO, and VSST.

6. When reporting "per-event" and/or "per-value stream" financial contributions to the ESC, if countermeasures are associated with the event or value stream, then check the "yes" box for the "CM in place?" question on the "Breakthrough Financial Contribution Monthly Summary Form".

7. Process Owner monitors progress of contributions and countermeasures, initiating further countermeasures if necessary.

January of 2010 the KCHC Behavioral Health team decided to explore the redesign of the Behavioral Health OPD revenue cycle. The current structure did not meet the newest regulatory requirements that would ensure compliance with delivery of care matched to coding and billing. The system was designed to fail. There were inconsistent methods in promulgating OPD appointments. Obtaining insurance authorizations prior to visits was unreliable and not reconciled. Accurate billing was jeopardized because of inaccurate coding and late visit closing. The target state for this RIE was focused on streamlining operations, creating standard work that would ultimately result in increased productivity, increased revenue, and improving patient and staff satisfaction.

The current state of disorganization took years to evolve. Lean allowed the organization to cut through the built-up silos in a short period of time. Frontline staff members mapped the real process. Waste was clearly identified as were the gaps of communication. New sustainable procedures were designed to meet users' needs. The new flow, with fewer handoffs between staff, elimination of redundant procedures, and real-time resolution of billing questions, created efficiencies that to date are maintained. Monthly monitoring has shown increased productivity, collectability, and patient/staff satisfaction. BHS believes the 30% additional cash realized in 2011 for the OPD is a direct result of the work performed in 2010.

Often, and in keeping with our balanced score card approach, achieving a clinical goal resulted in a financial benefit and vice versa. Direct observations (a ratio of one staff person to one patient, 1:1) are needed in certain circumstances to provide a safe environment for patients, yet they are costly and staff intensive. In calendar year 2010, the cost of 1:1 ratios at Kings County was calculated at $5.6 million. Decreasing the need for 1:1 ratios would result in freeing staff to perform needed clinical care for additional patients, which in turn would achieve the overall goal of recovery for the patient: an RIE was needed. Prework for the RIE revealed that there was a wide range of ordering patterns for the use of 1:1 ratios as there were no standard criteria used by providers. Documentation for the need of a 1:1 ratio was inconsistent, and the reassessment for the continued use was not dependable. The team of providers, nurses, and other allied staff reviewed the method of ordering (and reordering) direct observations. This RIE successfully incorporated an electronic solution to solve many of the communication needs that were previously buried in the patient record and not accessible to all appropriate staff members. One of the insights from this effort was that people in the best position to identify early changes in symptoms and behaviors had the least ownership of the milieu because there was no path for them to communicate directly to the decision maker. Training and empowering line staff, coupled with a visible whiteboard indicating which patients were on direct observation, decreased the use of 1:1 ratios. The financial impact of this RIE saved the institution $2,225,619 over 3 years. Figure 4.2 shows the dramatic decrease of 1:1 observations at Woodhull in 2010.

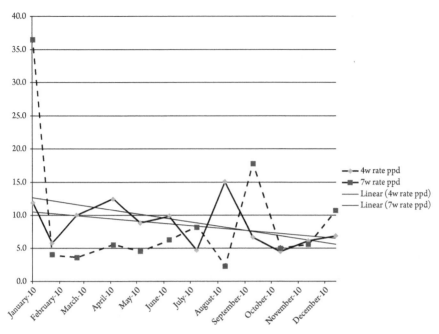

Figure 4.2 Decrease in 1:1 Observations. Source: Woodhull Medical and Mental Health Center 4W and 7W are inpatient psychiatry units. PPD = per patient day.

Queens Health-Care Network

Transforming any organization into a Lean/Breakthrough organization requires leaders to be effective strategic, financial, and process thinkers. This requires articulating and communicating a culture of continuous improvement driving change throughout all processes while pursuing a common vision. Long-term sustainment depends on the organization's leaders, managers, and supervisors actively participating in and supporting the new process while establishing key performance indicators (KPIs) to monitor progress.

SETTING FINANCIAL TARGETS USING HOSHIN KANRI

In 2009 the Queens Health Network became the first HHC network to introduce *hoshin kanri*, a lean planning and priority setting tool also known as policy deployment, to its senior leadership (see Box 4.2).

Subsequently, at the enterprise level, strategic priorities were identified for "must do, can't fail" initiatives that required alignment across the network and collaboration between previously siloed departments. These priorities were then further aligned to the TPOCs of each site so that implementation would occur through lean actions.

Box 4.2 **Hoshin Kanri**

The words "hoshin kanri" can be loosely translated from their Japanese origins as compass or direction and management or administration. It is commonly known as policy deployment and is a priority setting process that enables alignment of priorities between multiple levels of an organization. Elements include executive priority setting, identification of strategic initiatives, cascading these across an organization through a process of "catchball" to ensure understanding and decision making at appropriate levels, regular monitoring of incremental achievement, and establishment of timely countermeasures to ensure targets are reached. The hoshin kanri process requires interdisciplinary collaboration, horizontal and vertical alignment, and deselection of projects that do not contribute directly to the "critical few, must do, can't fail" initiatives. At HHC, hoshin kanri is applied from the corporate to the regional network and site level to support attainment of critical business goals. It takes time to acquire the discipline required to move from crisis management mode, in which chasing the problem of the day sucks time from strategic discussion and action, to a narrow focus on the incremental achievement of "breakthrough" priorities.

MEASURES AND COUNTERMEASURES

As hoshin kanri was implemented at Queens, the network enthusiastically moved toward achieving its goals. Deviations or barriers that were identified or impacted targets were addressed, and the owner of the work was required to establish countermeasures that would be implemented to bring the project back on track. Subgroups were also formed as appropriate to address these deviations. The results and steps taken were reported back at monthly reviews with senior leadership.

At first, the hoshin kanri process can be clunky as organizations become accustomed to this disciplined approach to priority setting and previously disparate activities are aligned and those that don't drive toward specifically articulated goals and objectives are considered for deselection. For Queens, for example, transitioning to a "24/7" hospital (one that could perform all necessary functions 7 days a week, 24 hours a day based on patient need) was a stretch for an organization that had less robust staffing on weekends and evenings. Set as a goal, with explicit expectations for achievement of incremental milestones and a certain end date, communication and prioritization were essential for success. In the monthly management meetings, it became difficult to maneuver around missed targets, and collaboration and persistence, as well as strong problem-solving competencies, became obvious as imperatives.

COMMUNICATION OF RESULTS THROUGHOUT THE ORGANIZATION

We discussed results that were being achieved through hoshin kanri on a regular basis throughout the network, including settings such as the Joint Labor Management meeting, where managers and labor staff met. Department Head and Town Hall meetings were additional forums where the information was also communicated. This communication helped to ensure that adequate stakeholder input was received and responded to and that surprises were limited.

INCREASING EFFICIENCIES AND DECREASING WASTE

The network was able to achieve some impressive results over the first 2 years of this collaborative work. In addition to bringing staff and leadership from the two hospitals in the network closer together, operational changes that had a direct impact on hoshin kanri targets were implemented across the network. Enhancing the role of the physician advisor, a relatively new type of position for the network, enabled clinicians to be on the units and in the emergency department on a full-time basis to solve problems and answer clinical questions related to hoshin kanri initiatives in real time. Weekend discharges increased, as did referrals for Cardiology from one site to the sister hospital, the regional center in the network.

INSIGHTS AND SUSTAINMENT

The network learned that it needed to improve communication about hoshin kanri to ensure that alignment across priorities, sites, and departments would be maintained. Balancing alignment between hoshin kanri goals and individual site TPOCs was essential to have the "boots on the ground" to move from planning to doing, to engage all tours, and to effectuate spread. The network achievements also benefited significantly from involving physicians and, as a result, encouraged the network to pull on additional physicians for this and other work. The Network has experienced an overall increase in physician participation and the development of embedded lean champions in clinical services. Various services have incrementally embraced lean concepts as a result of the attention given hoshin kanri initiatives. A3 Thinking and 6S workshops were introduced as a response to enlightened and invigorated staff. With the Queens Network leading the way, hoshin kanri was subsequently adopted at the enterprise level; HHC continues to work to cascaded it throughout the organization. Below are the strategic priorities represented in the 'Level 0 X-Matrix' (Box 4.3).

Any organization beginning a lean deployment should prepare itself for the many stages of improvement. At first the promise of real improvement is so enticing

---

Box 4.3 **HHC Fiscal Year 2014 Strategic Priorities**

- Achieve the Triple Aim (Better Care, Better Health, Lower Cost) while maintaining our mission.
- Achieve the integration of our delivery system necessary to succeed as an accountable care organization.
- Create an environment in which employees are safe, engaged, and enabled to contribute to the redesign of our system.

Source: NYCHHC FY14 Hoshin Kanri Level 0 X-Matrix.

---

that leaders rush to get results. The haste to implement leads to two critical failure modes. First is an underallocation of time to prepare for events, to analyze data, and to understand the value stream and the problem to be solved before beginning. Second is a failure to align the various improvements throughout the organization. Fortunately, there are many tools within lean to address these issues.

5

Lean in Behavioral Health

JOSEPH P. MERLINO, KRISTEN BAUMANN, AND JILL BOWEN

The previous chapters of this volume presented an introduction to lean and noted the successful application of lean principles and tools in both industry and health care. Lean was shown to be an effective methodology to improve staff development, safety, quality, efficiency, and fiscal return on investment. The principal strategy leading to these outcomes is quite simple: identification of unevenness in processes (variation), reduction of overburden of people or systems, and the elimination of waste wherever it is found within your system and returning the financial gains to the organization in a manner that supports the continued process of daily incremental performance improvement. It is important to note that lean is not about eliminating jobs but about repurposing staff roles to support continuous daily improvement.

The similarities in industry of needing to eliminate waste to increase efficiencies or to remove cumbersome steps that increase chances for error were recognized by medical professionals who adopted the tools and techniques of lean from industry and achieved equally impressive results. A resource for leaders in the fields of psychiatry, psychology, social work, behavioral health nursing, and the other behavioral health disciplines, lean offers methods to guide administrators and clinicians alike through the steps needed for successful transformative change. We believe that lean can work just as successfully in the field of behavioral health as it has in industry and general medicine. Safety metrics, from before and after lean's implementation, alone have demonstrated its effectiveness in behavioral health care (see Table 5.1).

The remainder of this volume explores a number of practical clinical challenges that you as a practitioner and/or as an administrator face and shows how lean can be of help to you and your organization across the full continuum of behavioral health care services so similar metrics can be achieved. Tools are demonstrated that can be used to assist leaders and practitioners with the creation and development of their vision, as well as the formulation of a plan of action for turning that vision into reality. Although this book is not intended to make you an expert in lean, nor to present lean as the only solution to your organizational transformation and quality

Table 5.1 **Safety True North Metrics for the Inpatient Services (205 beds) 2010 vs. 2012**

	Before	*After*
1:1 Orders	7,154	2,996
15-Day readmissions	163	107
IM orders	5,230	4,480
Restraint episodes	338	220

improvement, it seeks to demonstrate that lean can be a very useful tool for you and your organization.

At Kings County Hospital Center (KCHC), a large inner-city tertiary care safety-net public hospital located in an underserved area of Brooklyn, New York, we confront many of the same problems shared by other behavioral health care facilities, including budgetary constraints, a seemingly sicker patient population, and fewer community resources to partner with (see Figure 5.1).

Burning Platform/Reason for Action

Beyond the very real problems of budget, resources and capacity, we were confronted with a white hot "burning platform." Remember that the burning platform is the problem statement listed in Box 1 of the A3 (see Chapter 1) described earlier. It is the issue that gets you up and moving with a sense of urgency, as opposed to operating

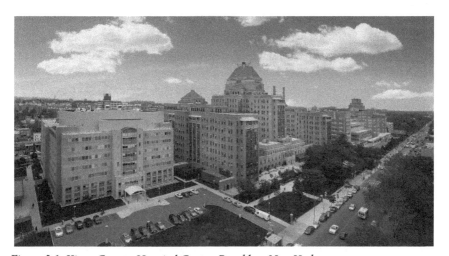

Figure 5.1 Kings County Hospital Center, Brooklyn, New York.

Kings County Hospital Center

New York City safety-net hospital; part of the Health & Hospitals Corporation
236 acute care behavioral health inpatient beds
3,000+ inpatient discharges per year
1,000+ detox discharges per year
8,000+ psychiatry emergency room visits per year
64,000 behavioral health outpatient visits per year
150,000+ chem/dep outpatient visits per year

---

in the usual routine day-to-day manner with the common issues with which we deal. Some background will help you appreciate our need for immediate improvement and total transformation and turnaround of our entire behavioral health system. A New York State agency, the "Mental Hygiene Legal Service (MHLS) provides legal services, advice, advocacy and assistance to persons receiving care or alleged to be in need of care at inpatient and community-based facilities for the mentally disabled. Created in 1964 and organized under Mental Hygiene Law article 47, MHLS represents such persons in judicial and administrative proceedings concerning admission, retention, transfer, treatment and guardianship. In addition to handling judicial proceedings, MHLS provides advice and representation regarding standards of care and other matters affecting the civil liberties of persons receiving care at facilities for the mentally disabled." [1] In 2007, MHLS together with the New York State Civil Liberties Union (CLU) increasingly raised concerns about the quality of care provided to the mentally ill at KCHC and they eventually sued the City of New York on May 2, 2007, citing numerous findings including overcrowded, unsanitary, and unsafe conditions where patients were routinely ignored and abused.

The United States Department of Justice (DOJ) also began monitoring conditions at the hospital in December 2007 because of complaints lodged by the New York CLU and others about improper conditions and treatment of the patients in the psychiatric division of the hospital. In June 2008, Esmin Green was taken to the comprehensive psychiatric emergency room in the old KCHC G building for a psychiatric evaluation with concerns that she needed psychiatric care and possible psychiatric hospitalization. She remained in the comprehensive psychiatric emergency program (CPEP) for many hours as she had refused examination for medical clearance to be admitted to the adult inpatient psychiatric unit. During the night tour she slid down off her chair onto the floor where she lay unattended despite staff walking by or looking into the area of the CPEP where she was confined. When staff did finally notice and attend to her she was in medical crisis and ultimately died. The sensational death of Ms. Esmin Green was captured on the hospital's security camera, and after it was leaked it was shown across the world. On January 15, 2009

Mental Hygiene Legal Service and Civil Liberties Union Concerns

Overcrowded psychiatry emergency room and inpatient units
"Dangerously unsanitary"
"Patients are routinely ignored and abused"
Patients are "subjected to illegal use of restraints and chemical injections,
neglect, and lack of proper services"

---

the DOJ issued its 58-page "findings letter," which detailed numerous violations of the Civil Rights of the Involuntarily Institutionalized Persons Act (CRIPA). This document was subdivided into nine substantive provisions:

1. Protection From Harm
2. Mental Health Care
3. Behavioral Management
4. Medical and Nursing Care
5. Quality Assurance/Performance Improvement
6. Fire and Life Safety
7. Discharge and Aftercare Planning
8. KCHC Hospital Police Policies, Procedures, and Practices
9. Training and Policy Manuals and Accountability

To address these findings and implement the transformational changes required, on February 2, 2009 new executive leadership was announced: a new Senior Vice President for the hospital and one of this volume's editors (JPM) as Administrator, or chief executive, for Behavioral Health Services.

A full year of legal negotiations followed between the New York City and Health & Hospitals Corporation (HHC) attorneys and the legal team for the DOJ and "Plaintiffs" (MHLS and the New York CLU and others), which produced two settlements with detailed plans of corrective actions (POCAS), one involving the DOJ and one for the MHLS and New York CLU. In total, there were more than 200 requirements for correction. Our job in Behavioral Health was to ensure the full and timely compliance with both court decrees. Yes, we had our burning platform. Box 1, check!

Initial State

Lean uses the A3 template to analyze a given problem and to identify solutions and a plan of action (see Figure 5.2). Our Initial State, Box 2 of the A3, described a huge mental health system operating in crisis mode, focused on putting out "fire" after

A3

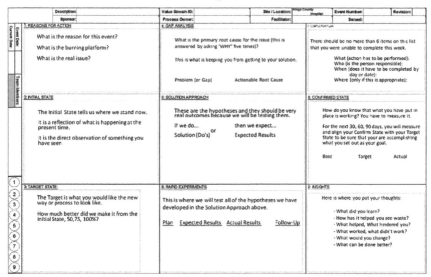

Figure 5.2 A3 thinking: Method for problem solving. The Lean A-3 Template.

"fire." We were operating our numerous services in seven old (mid-nineteenth—early twentieth century) buildings spread over a 44-acre campus. We were short-staffed and many of the staffs we had were transfers from other parts of the hospital and not familiar with or trained in working with psychiatric patients. Morale was low given the seemingly unending onslaught of negative publicity following the DOJ investigation and the sensationalized worldwide reporting of the death of Esmin Green. The culture was also largely complacent and dispirited. Some may describe the staff as exhibiting signs of learned helplessness/hopelessness. Staffs were largely not set up to be patient-centered or looking to empower patients, and many of the staffs of our services were not functioning as a coordinated interdisciplinary team. We lacked a leadership infrastructure and operated with an antiquated care delivery model. Inpatient units operated without "unit chiefs" and records were kept on paper without a system of chart review for quality and compliance. There were no interdisciplinary training programs in place that brought clinicians together with a unified vision of care delivery. And there was no model or hunger for change as a result of the learned helplessness that overtook many. Learned helplessness is the state that develops after repeatedly experiencing a toxic event from which one cannot escape. Eventually one gives up trying to escape even when the toxic event is removed.

Adding fuel to fire, we were on the heels of a scandal publicized worldwide, and patients and staff were frightened. Frightened by what the lawsuits would mean to our hospital and to us (some staffs were fired; others eventually arrested). Would the hospital be closed; would we be out of a job? We were also frightened not *for* our patients but *of* our patients who seemed more violent than most and often out of control, at least at this time in our trajectory. Assaults were high, as were serious injuries resulting from patient assaults on patients as well as patient assaults on staff. Triage in the psychiatric emergency room was suboptimal as was patient assessment, treatment, and aftercare planning. A true continuum of care was lacking with each service area siloed and disconnected from each other. Great variation existed, as evidenced by risk assessment on one inpatient unit not meaning the same as it did on other units. All of this led to poor outcomes for patients and staff alike as well as the legal actions that ensued.

Although increased focus began in 2007, regulatory and oversight scrutiny intensified so dramatically after the death of Ms. Esmin Green on June 19, 2008, and with the subsequent lawsuit and DOJ findings, that it became traumatizing to staff and the community. The feeling was one of loss of control, and the phrase, "Who's running the asylum?" captured the mood during that period. It was "us" versus "them," with the "them" seeming to be everyone: our patients, the community, hospital leadership, the media, and all the oversight agencies who took their turn descending on us with negative reviews and audits.

We were also fearful of successfully moving into our new behavioral health center. Frightened as to how we were going to move from the antiquated buildings we were in to the new behavioral health pavilion just completed without incidents and further negative publicity and regulatory scrutiny. Everyone recognized that having a new building, no matter how spectacular, did not in and of itself mean improved patient care, better outcomes, nor an energized and refocused staff. It should be noted that the planning for this $153 million, 360,000 square foot, seven-story structure began long before the problems in behavioral health at Kings County became national news, however ironic the timing of the completion of construction with the problems described above. The building of the new behavioral health center was part of a multiyear campus-wide redevelopment project at KCHC. Behavioral Health construction was the last phase of a four-phase project, although the timing came on the heels of the DOJ settlement agreement, it was notable and unfortunate that behavioral health was not part of an earlier rebuilding phase. Nevertheless, the modern behavioral health center symbolized a new era for behavioral health at Kings County and helped the staff and the community to visualize and contrast the "new" from the "old" behavioral health department.

Moving 230 inpatients plus all the patients in the psychiatric emergency room, along with the outpatient clinics, and all staff seemed daunting, especially given the "put out the fire" mode mentality we were all in while under the watchful eyes of the DOJ, the New York CLU and the New York MHLS, to say nothing of the New York City tabloids who were on constant watch for any misstep we might take, so they could sensationalize it with the goal of selling papers and recounting again and again the death of an ill woman in need of help who was neglected and left to die on our emergency room floor. We lost count of the number of times the video of Esmin Green dying on our floor was shown on television or reprinted in the newspapers.

Target State

Our goal, or target state (Box 3) seemed both obvious and at the same time impossible. The steps getting to that goal were many and included immediate, short-term and longer-term objectives that we mapped out through lean events, including visioning exercises and RIEs. These will be presented in more detail in the following chapters, but for now let's consider what was necessary to get us to that target state of substantial compliance with the requirements of the DOJ and the ending of their oversight, which would be concrete evidence of the successful transformation and turnaround of the behavioral health service of KCHC.

The optimism of staff involved in the first KCHC Behavioral Health Services (BHS) Lean Event was captured in their descriptions of what they saw as their goal—that is, their target state (see Staff Insights, next page).

The target state for Kings County Behavioral Health envisioned a strengthened CPEP as well as an inpatient and outpatient infrastructure staffed by caring, competent professionals. We wanted our new building to both symbolize as well as actualize a true transformation from the "snake pit" featured in the New York tabloids to the city's "flagship" public hospital. Quality and safety processes had to change, and outcomes had to be radically improved with leadership and line staff trained in the profession's best practices for assessment, diagnosis, treatment, and aftercare. The use of technology and data was seen as a tool to help us lead, manage, and deliver the needed improvement in quality care.

The overarching target goal was to achieve "substantial compliance" with the more than 200 provisions of the settlement with the DOJ and others. This designation was essential for the DOJ to end its monitoring of our facility. The DOJ estimated that based on their experience and the state of our institution that this would take 5 years at a minimum.

How Were We to Proceed?

First, we had to assemble a leadership team, who in turn needed to recruit adequate numbers of competent staff to join our ranks. We then had to ensure their training so that they both understood what was required by the POCAs and had the competencies to deliver what was required by the many policies and procedures that were recently reviewed, revised, and produced to attain compliance. Beyond understanding the POCA and DOJ requirements, our investment in training and proper staffing levels reflected the lean philosophy of focusing on human development first. We

---

Staff Insights

- There is a patient-centered, seamless flow of patients from reception to discharge. Wellness and recovery, with patient as collaborator, patient centeredness, and empowerment, as well as family empowerment, drive our service model. This includes the incorporation of peer counselors and evidence- based practices.
- Program operations will be transparent, data driven, and have clear lines of accountability.
- The CPEP attracts professionals who want to work with the KCHC patient population, who are compassionate team players, and who view themselves as part of a well-functioning, integrated system of emergency, outpatient, and inpatient care.
- Careful recruitment, ongoing training, and staff support are fundamental to the CPEP. The right people are in the right place. Staffs have, and take advantage of, opportunities for initial orientation to the KCHC model, ongoing learning, reflection, decompression, and renewal.
- Visual management and standard work are used throughout the CPEP to facilitate smooth operations and accommodate staffing changes and demand ebb and flow.
- Staff communication skills, including listening, with patients, families, and among staff across disciplines are excellent.
- The physical plant supports the therapeutic process. Workflows in the new building facilitate the effective employment of our service model, optimal utilization of space, and reflect respect for patients, family, and staff.
- The physical plant supports the therapeutic process. Workflows in the new building facilitate the effective employment of our service model, optimal utilization of space, and reflect respect for patients, family, and staff.

---

had to really decide whether we had the right people, in the right place, doing the right job. Further, are we giving these people all the tools, opportunities, and support they need to achieve our goals?

As the senior team was assembled, every former clinical discipline director eventually was replaced with new leaders. Surprisingly, the negative publicity about Kings County seemed to attract, not deter, exceptional leaders and staff, especially when during interviews the senior team displayed openness and a lack of defensiveness about the past, the current challenges and the vast potential for the Behavioral Health Service's future. It was gratifying to hear the newly recruited leadership speak passionately about their desire to join the challenge of redefining the mental health care system for a population as large as central Brooklyn, seeing it as a once-in-a-career opportunity. Most of our new leadership came from other inner-city hospitals and were familiar with the many challenges presented in such settings. With the addition of resources mandated by the DOJ, these leaders saw the opportunity to remake a behavioral health department in accordance with their vision of how it should be done right, benefitting the patients, the community, and the staff.

Once assembled, the new leadership team needed to rebuild the "old psychiatric hospital" from the ground up and to create the systems and processes to ensure operations that provided a safe setting for patients and staff alike so that best practices of care could be developed and competently delivered. We have learned that, even if you invest in the right number of sufficient staff, if your processes are faulty, then your people will fail. Ultimately, we needed to integrate each of the many fragmented services into one seamless continuum of care that improved access to care and delivered state of the art care to our consumer-partners in a timely and cost-effective way. This was referred to as achieving the "triple aim"—namely, better health, better quality care, and reduced overall cost. This would hopefully result in the DOJ finding us in substantial compliance and end their oversight of Kings County Hospital Center Behavioral Health Services. Then, having the tools, experience, and mentoring to achieve our gains, we would be able to independently sustain those gains while continuing to add value, decrease waste, and continuously improve performance and outcomes. In other words, to become the Center of Excellence that the DOJ, our community, and New York's HHC expected of us—and this within a 5-year period!

Gap Analysis

SCOPE OF EVENT: FOCUS ON EMERGENCY ROOM OR TAKE ON ENTIRE DEPARTMENT?

To state the obvious, there were numerous gaps between the current and target states that needed to be addressed and overcome. But with so many problems and a system so large, we weren't sure how or where to start. A major concern was for patient and staff safety. Believing that therapy could not occur unless both patients and staff felt safe, overall safety became priority number one. Some of the metrics used to monitor safety are demonstrated in Table 5.2 and included the number of serious (that is state reportable) incidents, use of physical restraints, and administration of intramuscular injections for aggressiveness. Early readmission to hospital within 15 days of discharge was also monitored. Table 5.3 shows that sustained improvement has occurred in most areas.

The task seemed daunting, overwhelming, and at times frankly impossible. During the period we were confronting these issues at Kings County, our parent corporation, the New York City HHC, was in the process of introducing the lean

Table 5.2 **A3 Box 8 Confirmed State Restrictive Interventions RIE Safety Metrics**

Indicator	Metric	Baseline	Target
Safety	Incidents	6 NIMERS reportable incidents	Good = 5 Very Good = 4 Outstanding = 3
Safety	Restraint	Adult 0.142 per 100 patient days	Good = 071 Very Good =. 066 Outstanding =. 042
Quality	Stat Psychotropic IMs	Adult Rate = 10 per 100 days	Good= 8 Very Good = 7 Outstanding = 5
Safety/ Quality	Recidivism	Adult & Child 15-day readmission rate = 6.9%	Good = 6% Very Good = 5.5% Outstanding = 5%

way of thinking and problem solving throughout its 11 hospitals. In 2008 lean had not yet made its way to Kings County. However, in light of the challenges of our burning platform, including the unique opportunity that moving into a new hospital building afforded, HHC's corporate leadership responded to our "pull" by bringing lean methodology to our hospital earlier than originally planned, and our behavioral health service became the newest HHC lean "value stream."

In lean terminology, the entire service line of the behavioral health division of Kings County Hospital, about one-third of the entire hospital complex, was identified as a "value stream." A value stream encompasses all the activities that are required within an organization to deliver a specific service. Behavioral health, especially in hospital-based settings, sometimes is organized so that the full range of the continuum of care falls under one administrative umbrella. In these organizations, psychiatric emergency services, inpatient services, ambulatory services, and chemical dependency services—for adults as well as adolescents and children—all fall within the same department and under the same overall clinical and administrative leadership. For example, nursing, social work, and even the medical teams reported to the CEO of Behavioral Health so that service delivery could be facilitated with less bureaucracy and in a more integrated fashion; all of this is consistent with the lean principles of decreased waste and improved quality.

Another reason for considering all of behavioral health as one integrated value stream was that patients move through the many different parts of our continuum of care during their treatment and recovery, often during different stages of their lives. As a result, many of our patients are known across our system from previous contact with one or another of our programs. In planning lean events, this made it

Table 5.3 **Visual Management Grid Showing Sustained Improvement: Goal Met *Goal not met***

	Metric	Baseline	Target	7/13/10	8/10/1D	9/10/10	10/10/10	11/9/10	12/7/10	1/7/11	2/7/11	3/7/11
s	Incidents All Units	6 NIMERS reportable incidents	Good = 5 Very Good = 4 Outstanding = 3	5 NIMERS GOOD	3 NIMERS OUT-STANDING	6 NIMERS GOOD	2 NIMERS OUT-STANDING	3 NIMERS OUT-STANDING	1 NIMERS OUT-STANDING	**10 NIMERS**	6 NIMERS GOOD	5 NIMERS GOOD
s	Restraint All Units	Adult 0.142 per 100 pt days	Good = .090 Very Good = .066 Outstanding = .042 Corporate average: Adult 0.1	**.386**	.087 GOOD	**.538**	**.208**	**.290**	**.324** Intervention BST early intervention new RN leadership: unit specific training; & pilot units performing better!	**.394** Intervention BST early intervention 3W &7W; & pilot units performing better!	059 OUT-STANDING Intervention STANDING	**.409**
Q	Stat psychotropic IMs All units	Adult Rate = 10 Per 100 days	Good = 9 Very Good = 8 Outstanding = 7	**9.8**	8 VERY GOOD	8 VERY GOOD	8 VERY GOOD	6 OUTSTAN	5.4 OUTSTAN	5.6 OUTSTAN	5.59 OUT-STANDING	5.9 OUT-STANDING
S / Q	Recidivism All units	Adult & Child 15-day Readmission rate = 6.9%	Goods = 6% Very Good= 5.5% Outstanding = 5%	**Adult=7%** Child 4% OUT-STANDING	**Adult=6.6%** Child 2.6% OUT-STANDING	**Adult=7.4%** Child 0% OUT-STANDING	Adult=3.2% OUTSTAN Child 3.2% OUT-STANDING	Adult=1.2% OUTSTAN Child 1.5% OUT-STANDING	Adult = 6.1% GOOD Child = 3.7% OUT-STANDING	Adult = 6.2% GOOD Child = 2.9% OUT-STANDING	Adult = 3.2% OUTSTAN Child = 2.9% OUT-STANDING	Adult =4.2% OUT-STANDING **Child = 6.6%**

both easier to address issues across the continuum, yet also more difficult because we had to delineate a scope for each lean event that was manageable trying to avoid "scope creep"—that is, not taking on more than can be effectively "fixed" during a lean event and subsequently sustained.

STRATEGY: LONG-TERM VERSUS MONTH-TO-MONTH

The challenge of scope, how much of the many gaps between current and target states to tackle and when, needed to be confronted in preparing each lean event and strategic decisions made by the BHS lean steering committee. A tension always existed between our desire to take on all we believed needed fixing versus what could realistically be achieved within the timeframe of each lean event (e.g., 4.5 days for a RIE). Change in culture and practice, particularly in public hospitals and other community psychiatry settings, is not known for its speediness—thus the urgency to improve quickly in multiple areas posed the risk of taking on too broad a scope at a given time. The danger in this was not succeeding in implementation and sustainment, thus frustrating staff at best and having the entire lean process lose credibility at worst. We had to learn to plan for making changes in both depth and breadth of scope using various lean tools.

Value Stream Analysis

This is a strategic planning event that helps translate areas identified to be problematic in a service into an actionable plan. The process forces leaders to make connections through a large system to understand how customers, suppliers, patients, staff, and information flow through a system. Often care has many detours and dead ends in the approach to care—a value stream analysis (VSA) hopes to establish a delivery system that enables flow rather than hinder flow through different levels of care.

Typically VSAs are looking at your next 12 months and establishing a sequence of 12 RIEs and less than six projects that build on one another to achieve the goals established in the VSA. Most organizations look at the short term and solve the crisis of the month. VSAs help define for people in concrete terms (through consensus building and data) the long-term plans and how a group can get there. Leadership sets a plan of action for the year, giving focus to their staff as to what the priorities are for that given time frame.

Rapid Improvement Events

This is not a planning event but a doing event. What we mean by this is we take pieces of our system (identified in the VSA) and look at them under a magnifying glass and make change happen by the week's end. Central to this process is that RIE teams are made up of staff from those areas focused on to encourage staff to become better problem solvers and even stakeholders. They analyze a specific problem, determine its root cause, and through rapid experiments work toward a 50% improvement by the end of the 4.5-day event.

Conducting visioning events once a year helped us look at yearly strategic plans—the big picture at the 30,000-foot level, whereas RIEs taught us to drill an "inch wide and a mile deep," getting deep into the weeds to solve problems. Along with project planning these visioning events helped us articulate a vision and common goals for staff and leaders to work toward together. This is referred to in lean as alignment.

NO REAL SYSTEM FOR CHANGE

When HHC headquarters offered to bring and support lean at Kings County to bring our burning platform under control, we grabbed at the opportunity of leading by lean. What does it mean to "lead with lean?" Leading with lean means leading with a vision: a unifying vision that helps to steer the direction of the organization toward attaining its key, or "true north," metrics. Heading true north toward a vision clearly communicated by leadership provides a clear goal and helps keep the multiple lean initiatives aligned, particularly important in behavioral health settings with its multiple service areas and departments. To set the true north metrics and to guide the overall process of transformation, a lean value stream steering committee is essential.

Lean is one of a number of process improvement methodologies. HHC chose lean because the "fit" felt better than other processes (e.g., Six Sigma). We are not advocating that you choose lean over other processes, but we are urging you to select one and stay with it. Leading with a lean vision is different than other efficiency methodologies because, executed correctly, it fundamentally changes the culture of the organization in parallel with changing processes focusing on a specific value stream, adding value to the end-user, with a focus on eliminating waste. In *The Lean Turnaround*, Byrne notes, "In fact, the modern management approach tends to focus on everything but the value-adding activities when looking to improve the company's results."[2] Changing the hearts and minds through the course of the journey, by directly engaging people in the gemba (the actual work site) with a learn-by-doing approach, facilitates culture shift to occur.

This sets lean apart from other transformation methodologies—for example, Six Sigma. A pure Six Sigma approach requires highly trained engineering types to complete statistical modeling through a software system, such as Minitab. The modeling is then used to show variation and suggest changes to a process. The changes are deployed and measured to monitor the effectiveness of those changes toward eliminating variation. Although lean is also a very data-driven efficiency model, a pure lean approach is based on training the people that are directly engaged with completing the work in a given process, with simple tools and approaches such as a waste, walk, and time observations, to train their eyes to see waste in their respective processes. The direct observations of the process are then compared to process output data, such as productivity, to brainstorm suggested changes to the process that will eliminate the observed waste. The changes are tested, deployed, and measured for effectiveness of the changes toward eliminating waste.

Lean also differs in subtle but critical ways, from approaches such as "Management by Objectives (MBO) or other methods that use a cascading goals process to communicate corporate objectives and develop business unit-level means of achieving them."[3] These differences include the following:

- True north metrics chosen by an intensive process of data gathering and consensus building
- Collaboration and give-and-take as the goals are cascaded down through the organization
- Engagement of all levels of the organization[4]

The steering committee is a central component of the leadership structure and an integral part of planning events, defining scope, monitoring the implemented initiatives for sustainment, and, above all, removing obstacles, all with the aim of moving the organization toward that ultimate vision; in our case, substantial compliance with the 200-plus requirements of the DOJ. In our very large behavioral health department, approximating the size and scope of five separate departments (emergency services, inpatient services, ambulatory services, pediatrics, and medical), plus chemical dependency, this structure is particularly critical to alignment of events aiming in the same direction of true north and ultimately, overall success. Figure 5.3 shows the connections between the A3 visioning events, the lean steering committee at the value stream, and at the executive enterprise levels.

Regardless of the size of your behavioral health organization, however, a guiding vision and the organizational structure of the steering committee is essential for keeping your initiatives aligned and ensuring that they contribute to the overall vision and direction of the organization as a whole and that of the specific value stream (see Figure 5.4).

Like the officers at the helm of a ship, the steering committee sets overall direction including parameters and high-level project guidance as it steers the value stream in the direction of true north. The steering committee reviews the status of milestones using metrics and approves resource requirements, facilitating the involvement of various hospital departments like facilities, finance, information technology, etc. It represents the interests of critical stakeholders and is responsible for providing advice and recommendations to the various lean teams working on RIEs or projects. This team generally includes clinical and administrative leadership across behavioral health services, led by the value stream's executive sponsor. This steering committee leader is typically the chief executive officer or other senior executive who is ultimately responsible for championing and signing off on

Roles and Linkages

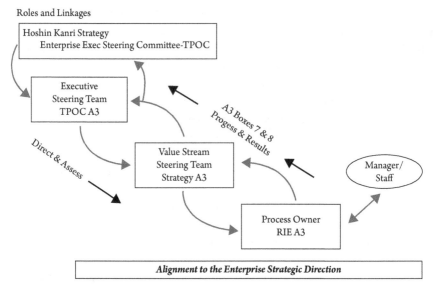

Figure 5.3 Lean infrastructure.

Breakthrough Improvement System

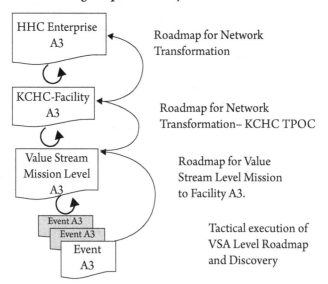

Figure 5.4 Lean Alignment.

the plans for change in an organization and who keeps initiatives aligned with the larger organization's strategy and true north metrics, as well as provides leadership on culture change and adherence to organizational values. He or she also sits on the hospital-wide executive steering committee for lean.

SYSTEMS OF COMMUNICATION FOR CHANGE

Recall that a crucial tool for focusing the team and planning the events that would guide the transformation activities is called a "visioning event." A visioning event is a highly interactive senior-level group collaboration designed to stimulate discussion and the exchange of ideas about the future direction of the organization. Visioning sessions are extremely valuable during the process of preparing for events. Participants work as a team to identify areas for improvement and provide an important baseline for developing formal projects, and "just-do-its" (JDIs).

This was the laboratory where the elucidation of vision, designation of scope, and organization of the huge undertaking of transforming BHS at KCHC took place. Through this process the gaps we needed to confront were revealed including: increasing the number and skills of staff in BHS, having them work as an effective interdisciplinary team, conversion of the culture of complacency into one of engagement, integration of silos into a seamless continuum of care, and conversion of the medical model into a patient-centered wellness and recovery model—to name some of the most critical.

Now that the gaps from initial state to ideal state were identified, the work of how to close those gaps was tackled. This occurs in Box 5 of the A3 and is called the "solution approach."

Solution Approach

The first visioning event at KCHC BHS occurred November 2008. This was approximately 5 months after the death of Ms. Green and about 3 months prior to moving into the new behavioral health facility. Since our CPEP was a major focal point of both the Green tragedy and the lawsuits, our first foray into using lean methodology to guide our transformation was focused there. The CPEP in the old "G building" was small (one-third the size of the new one) and often overcrowded (sometimes with a census of 40–50) with limited space for movement of either patients or staff. Key stakeholders were chosen to kick-off the lean journey for KCHC BHS. All were novices to the lean process and all understood the clear and pressing mandates for rapid and substantial improvement. Successful change in our CPEP, it was hoped, would lead the true transformation of our entire system of behavioral health care.

Although, as you will see, the tools and techniques of lean became essential to our transformation, lean was introduced in a less gradual and incremental manner than is usual for an organization. Gradual introduction helps an organization to learn about the process of lean, begin to learn the language as a group, and to have the time to anticipate that a new approach is coming before they dive into its use. We did not have that luxury. Because of the intensity of our burning platform, we needed to do all of those steps simultaneously. We needed to make change happen, and fast.

The first visioning event was an education in itself. A visioning event brings awareness of the areas needing improvement to the fore and provides tools for setting events into motion to realize the vision of making those improvements and having them stick. Our staff had to learn the terminology of lean, as well as grasp a beginning understanding of how lean tools had been applied in other health care settings and how these might prove helpful to us. This was a "hit the ground-running, learn as you go" event that catapulted us forward on our lean journey. The feeling was very much one of "sink or swim; do or die."

Leading by lean also means visibility and transparency to all staff. You cannot lead by lean from behind a desk. The leadership needs to be visible, modeling, redirecting, and supporting the staff. With lean, this occurs by leadership walking the gemba, or the place where the work is done. John Toussaint of ThedaCare has noted, "Senior leadership of most companies spend shockingly little time... [a]t Toyota, on the other hand, going to the gemba meant assisting operations: looking for problems or improvement opportunities and finding out what workers need to stay on target. It means getting to know, first hand, the issues facing front-line workers and helping to work out solutions. It means learning, not teaching and telling."[5]

Liker and Convis, in their book, *The Toyota Way to Lean Leadership*, stress that the success and sustainment of a lean approach depends not on the technique but on the leadership and its development throughout the organization. "Few companies see this connection between Toyota leadership and the company's exceptional results... [b]ut replicating Toyota's technical systems without understanding their source... has largely proved futile."[6] That "source" is the culture in which all staff are partners working with management across the organization (horizontally, not vertically in silos) and in which its leaders see "self-development and training others as the only possible path, not only for finding the right solution for the problem at hand, but for constantly and consistently improving performance day after day."[4] Liker and Convis see the approach needed for lean to be successful as akin to losing weight that requires a lifestyle change and commitment, not a crash diet, for sustained success.

The information learned and metric targets set needed to be visible to all staff along with a display of our progress and/or obstacles to meeting our goals. A useful way to achieve this is by doing "gemba (actual site of the work) walks" and having "mission control" displays in the gemba so staff could conveniently see and always be a partner in what was happening. The mission control displays portrayed graphs and other visuals simply communicating progress or lack thereof along with corrective actions, or countermeasures, to attain the targeted metrics.

We learned how lean engages staff, in part, by bringing line staff front and center into the various improvement events. The spread of lean knowledge among line staff was itself a metric monitored to help measure culture change and transformation in the organization. Our goal was to increase the number of staff involved in some way with lean by 20% per year, not simply in hearing about lean but by actually being involved directly in lean events like RIEs.

Initially we used lean in planning for the first few months on the operations of the CPEP, with some attention to the general planning for the move of our services into the new "R" building from the several buildings from which we were currently operating. Most of our services to be moved resided in the old "G" building. Within the next 2 months, "standard work" for CPEP staff, roles, and functions as well as plans to support the move from the G to the R buildings would be underway. Remember that standard work is the written-down steps needed to be consistently followed to ensure that the lessons learned from lean events are followed without variation thus ensuring the gains achieved in the experiments of the events would be reliably replicated going forward. Lean events uncover waste and develop ways to eliminate that waste and add value to our patients and to our staff. Standard work memorializes this and fosters the sustainment of improvements.

Measuring compliance with standard work as well as keeping track of your goals and targets is where the use of metrics is so important. Metrics in lean are the foundation of the data analysis and help you to keep track of the impact of the plans set in motion in a formal way. Metrics are variables that are measured and monitored and used to detect errors or variation. These are then evaluated and analyzed serving to guide decisions that lead to further improvements.

An organization's true north metrics guide its strategic and philosophical vision. They are grouped into the general categories of Human Development, Quality/Safety, Timeliness, Cost, and Growth and Development. These metrics and other key information need to be clearly and simply displayed throughout the organization as tools for visual management. Often less is more as in using a simple bar graph to illustrate the increase or decrease in attaining a particular metric with a simple explanatory box beneath the graph, including any course-correcting measures to be taken.

The focus in CPEP initially was on the true north metrics of Quality and Safety, and our lean events started right up front at the process of clinical triage. It was agreed that triage metrics would be a major focus because a large part of the lawsuit by the MHLS had to do with timeliness of various processes, like triage, in the CPEP. Decreasing triage times was considered essential for improving the experience of the patient and reducing overall waiting time for assessment, treatment, and disposition in the CPEP. Our premise was that decreasing triage time would result in improving quality of care by more quickly assessing, diagnosing, and beginning treatment of our patients.

The overcrowding of the CPEP was also highlighted in the lawsuits as a significant contributor to the problems faced at KCHC. The flow of patients through our system began with entry into CPEP and with the triage process itself. Our vision was for the patient to enter the CPEP where he/she would be met and welcomed by staff including a nurse, doctor, and peer (former behavioral health patient now working as part of the interdisciplinary team) and to minimize the total number of steps needed before a patient got to reach triage. There were two triages that had been created in such a way as to avoid duplication while enhancing safety and timeliness: the traditional one for nurses and a second one for psychiatrists. Safety would be improved by improving the triage process: triage entailed quickly assigning the appropriate level of care needed by the patient and to ensure that the patient was able to see a psychiatrist within a short period of time from entry into the CPEP. The nursing triage was to be done within 30 minutes and the psychiatric triage within 60 minutes of a patient's presentation (see Figure 5.5).

Once the RIE took place, standards of work were developed and written for each step in the patient's flow to ensure that safe, high-quality triage activities occurred for all who entered the CPEP. It was agreed in the visioning event that the RIE and standard work training for CPEP would take place in the yet to be occupied new R building CPEP to allow the staff to get into the new space, familiarize themselves

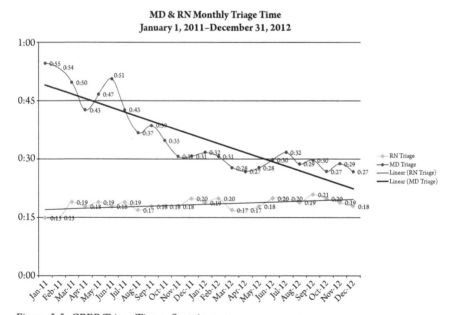

Figure 5.5 CPEP Triage Times: Sustainment.

with it, and to practice the standard work in the actual space where it would soon be provided.

As noted, leading by lean means being visible in the space where the work takes place, the "gemba." Having both leadership and line staff working together in what would become the new gemba of the CPEP began to set the tone of the new approach emphasizing respect, collaboration, and teamwork. Visual management tools were especially helpful (see Figure 5.6). These included simple illustrations to quickly show staff in a given work area how they were doing on the lean task(s) specific to them. This is similar to the cartoon of a thermometer often used to display how a fund drive is doing in terms of reaching its goal. This is a visual management tool. Staff should only need a few seconds to look at the visual to grasp whether or not they are succeeding. Where goals are off course, the corrective measures are explained on the visual board. The "mission control" room/area, where many visuals are displayed for the lean steering committee, depicts these in more detail than the simple and focused ones posted in specific work areas.

In addition to posting written standards of work in the gemba, flow diagrams were also displayed so that all CPEP staff could easily see what was supposed to happen and whether or not it was happening (see Figure 5.7). A sample of the flow process was enacted and videotaped to help staff understand the new plan for patient flow and the needed processes to achieve this for the CPEP. One of the earliest metrics studied was triage time. The data on nursing and psychiatric triage times have been tracked since 2009 and is a lean success story, with achievement and sustainment now longer than 3 years.

Lean helped us determine what was important for success, what we needed to do, and how to measure it, achieve it, and sustain it. George Koenigsaecker, in

Visual Management Tool

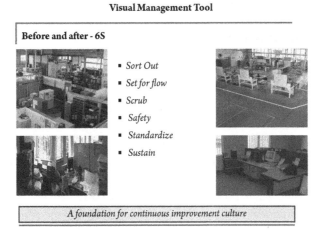

Figure 5.6 Visual Management Tool: "6 S".

One-Piece Flow

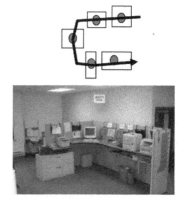

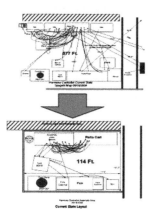

- Value Add right next to each other
- No Waiting, Continuous Flow
- 1 By 1

Figure 5.7 One Piece Flow.

Leading the Lean Enterprise Transformation, outlines the process by which lean does this so well. He describes the "building blocks" of lean culture as[7] :

Serve the customer
Seek what's right or "active honesty"
Decide carefully, implement quickly
Candidly admit imperfections
Speak honestly and with deep respect
Go, see, and listen to learn
Deliver on meaningful challenges
Be a mentor and a role model

This is just a sample of the CPEP story. You will read more about our work in the CPEP in Chapter Seven, "Lean and Inpatient Psychiatry."

Moving From the Old Hospital to the New

Let's now look at another early challenge: the process of moving the behavioral health hospital from its old home to its new one. As to the massive move itself from multiple buildings across 44 acres to one multistoried building, involving acute inpatient and emergency patients, outpatient clinics and day programs, as well as interagency coordination needed, the application of lean to the planning was very helpful. As a result of lean preparation focusing on patient flow and workflow, gaps, and standard work, the move went off amazingly well and truly without a hitch. The A3 thinking that is part and parcel of lean methodology helped us to identify significant gaps in areas that needed coordination and solutions in planning the big move. Because the move occurred early in our lean journey, we were still very new to these techniques, but the focus of identifying the target state and analyzing the gaps in the initial proposal facilitated several iterations of the plans so that identified gaps could be closed proactively. The major gap identified was the absence of, and the clear need for, several very well-coordinated efforts. Multiple departments within Kings County would be involved, including Behavioral Health, Medicine, Facilities Management, Transport, and Hospital Police, as well as outside agencies such as New York's emergency medical services (which operated the city ambulances), the New York City Police Department, the Board of Education, the State Office of Mental Health, and the New York Department of Health. Huddles with key stakeholders and the use of visual management tools again helped to ensure good communication and served to simplify an otherwise complex undertaking.

In our A3 analysis, one of the steps identified was the need to coordinate the various activities to make certain that interdependent systems within Behavioral Health were not left on their own. For example, the CPEP and one of the six adult inpatient units moved over to the new building first so that patients who were admitted would have a bed ready in the same building rather than having to be admitted to the old building only later to be moved to the new building. Remember the goal of all lean endeavors is to identify and eliminate waste, including repeating steps or processes. Moving one inpatient unit simultaneously with the CPEP eliminated rework and wasted time and energy and of course eliminated the avoidable inconvenience to our patients. By bringing half the patients from this receiving unit over, half the beds were left empty and available for new admissions from the CPEP. Additionally, the staff were able to practice making the move on a smaller and more manageable scale, increasing our chances for a smooth transition. The first patients selected to be moved were those assessed as most psychiatrically and medically stable. On the following day, other inpatient units moved—one unit at a time; this is the lean concept of "one piece flow." The coordinated plans involved three teams to support the patient transition—one team helping to get patients ready in the old G building, a second team positioned along the route to be traveled and in the vans with the patients to ensure appropriate care and calm, and the third team stationed physically on the new receiving units in the R building to welcome patients as they arrived and to assist them in settling into their new rooms and orienting them to the new unit.

The development of and adherence to standard work ensured that all staff on the three teams knew their roles well and could work together in a unified and seamless manner. Notably, the establishment of this standard work unexpectedly served us well during New York City's emergency evacuation, during Hurricane Irene in 2011, of one of Brooklyn's other hospitals, Coney Island Hospital, to KCHC. Fears of major flooding resulted in the transfer of a full psychiatric unit from Coney Island Hospital to the KCHC R Building. This transfer used the same standard of work, and again, the transfer was flawless! These same plans were once again relied on as we prepared yet again for the second hurricane in 2 years, Hurricane Sandy in 2012, when both Coney Island Hospital and Bellevue Hospital Center were evacuated and closed for prolong periods of time. Several of their patients were evacuated to the KCHC BHS.

The simultaneous closing of the old CPEP, heretofore the major receiving psychiatric service for Brooklyn, and the opening of the new CPEP required extensive coordination among KCHC, New York City's Emergency Medical Services, and other voluntary and private ambulance services. The plan was for sufficient lead time to be built into the system, the right people identified and in the loop to conduct the transition, and all communication to be organized and coordinated so that only one CPEP was in operation at a time. This went off like clockwork, with EMS informed and smoothly transitioning the transport of patients to the new R CPEP, and no longer to G. Had this not been as well planned and coordinated, patients could have been brought to a closed psychiatric emergency room, creating more waste of time, delayed treatment, and potentially harmful outcomes. One could almost hear a collective sigh of relief by New York's emergency services when this went off so smoothly!

The child and adolescent services coordinated with the board of education so that the inpatient schools moved from G to R as the children moved. The outpatient services also moved easily with a good deal of effort made to provide clear information to patients and the community so all knew where they were to go and when. Once again, visual tools were helpful in this regard, showing staff and patients what was happening and when and what they were to do to get to the correct place at the correct time. Eliminating waste proved highly useful in decreasing confusion and increasing efficiency in the use of time and the elimination of the need for corrective actions or rework.

So the move itself, supported by lean techniques facilitating the planning, went well. Once in the new R building, however, the highly technological state-of-the-art building did not work as planned. Although everything from computer systems to secured swipe-card entries had worked before the move, once all were in place they started failing in a rather dramatic manner. Although the best laid plans often go astray, this was indeed an interesting and challenging time.

The usefulness of the previously developed and practiced standards of work that were put into effect was evident and seemed a godsend during this crisis period. The use of huddles with key stakeholders served to keep clear lines of communication open. Back-up plans in the event of technological failures were in place and operationalized, including specifics as to what to do in the event of specific failures such as phones not working or computerized medication order systems not working. There were processes in place to provide the necessary information about medication ordering in alternate ways and there were particular phones on the units that were especially hard-wired for use in emergencies, as well as the availability of cell phones. The highly technological swipe-entry mechanisms also had key overrides that were available to staff on the units. The availability of these standards of work for back-up systems, improved communication, and processes that had been developed with input from key stakeholders helped restore some calm during this very stressful next storm. Once again, A3 thinking helped to organize us to confront these unanticipated facility's failures when they occurred and also taught us to be wary of the issue of computer overload in the event of future massive moves requiring high-tech support. The kinks eventually did get worked out of the system as the overloading of the computerized systems became evident and was corrected with additional hardware and software.

Spreading Lean to Other Areas of Care

Having now successfully relocated and with a reasonable sense of comfort that our CPEP was functioning as planned, by May 2009 the BHS wanted to take on its next challenge. More new leadership had come on board in the previous months, staff had adapted well to the new building, and the DOJ and plaintiff mandates continued to unfold with each of their subsequent compliance visits every 6 months.

It became apparent that for culture change to occur on this order of magnitude, the new leadership team needed to forge a new vision for KCHC BHS. The urgency of the situation in 2008's visioning, which focused on the hospital move and the opening of the new CPEP, did not provide for an overall comprehensive look at the department as a whole, which should have been the first visioning event in more usual scenarios and is what you are advised to do! Recall that earlier it was noted that the way we started with lean at Kings County was not what was typically recommended. It is advisable to wade into the waters of lean, not jump head first into the deep end, as we felt we had to do.

In the 2009 visioning event, the team sought to include the entire continuum of care beyond CPEP, taking lean next to the inpatient and outpatient services. This "30,000-foot view" was hopeful, if massive in scope, and reflected the growing sense of opportunity and energy that the new leadership brought to bear. Recall that the purpose of a VSA is to identify the specific activities occurring along an entire value stream. This results in seeing waste, as well as opportunity, and encourages sharing of vision, communication, and predicting results with the use of measured metrics over time. The VSA for Behavioral Health at this point in time was an extremely helpful analysis used to create an action plan for improvement, which sought to incorporate known best practices while simultaneously creating new best practices along our clinical continuum of care from CPEP to the inpatient division and on to the outpatient clinics ending in successful reintegration back into the community in some stage of wellness and recovery as defined by the recipient of care.

The solution approach to closing the gap between the then current state and the target state at that time was to embrace the continuum of care in a patient-centered manner, so that staff moved with the patients and that teams were not wedded to a particular service area like inpatient or outpatient. This would require that the admitting team in the CPEP would essentially follow the patient they admitted throughout his/her treatment course from point of entry into our system to time of discharge, which could occur months to several years later. Although exciting, and serving to forge the new leadership into an effective team, this was a scope that it was quickly recognized needed to be trimmed back, way back! And it was.

Recall that scope defines what is covered and what is not within a particular event and time period. The scope is the boundary of what a project or an event will focus on. Scope is critical so that what *needs* to be achieved *can* be achieved in the time allotted. A vision can be too grand to realize within a realistic period of time and will lead to unsuccessful implementation or sustainment of the improvements sought. This also leads to staff demoralization and a sense of futility that so much has to be done and that it can't possibly be achieved in the time allotted. This is not the message we want staff to receive.

Rather, lean encourages continuous incremental advancement so that improvements are attainable, as well as sustainable, with each building on the success of another. We recognized, when we came to our senses and with the guidance of our sensei, that the entire continuum of care would be too massive to transform all at once. In the words of our sensei, "You can't boil the ocean." The decision was made that our initial focus, measured by clearly identified metrics, was to remain on the acute care services (CPEP/emergency and inpatient divisions) for the time being. We learned that overreach is not an uncommon problem as organizations prepare the scope of their events, especially early in their journey. Often "too much is bitten off" too early, reflecting leadership's hope of making quick changes. Although noble in spirit, it is best to take on a scope of transformation that can be achieved and sustained, permitting success to breed future success. Remember, lean is about continuous *incremental* improvement that leads to radical overall transformation. The steering committee keeps its "pedal to the metal" while keeping one eye on the road ahead and the other on the rear view mirror.

Using the Vertical Value Stream Map

Within a few months a third visioning event, this time a vertical value stream mapping (VVSM) was employed to help sort out priorities in terms of which areas to tackle and when, while keeping the vision of overall transformation alive and sustaining the gains already made.

A VVSM is a drawing that depicts the flow of the processes and information along a value stream. For the behavioral health value stream, this meant looking at the different ways in which patients moved or flowed through our continuum of services, as well as the flow of staff communication and activity as they performed the necessary functions for providing direct care and support services (see Figure 5.8). This visual "map" displays the linked series of processes that shows how a full service flows from its starting point until it ultimately gets into the hands of the customer.

A VVSM helps to organize particularly complex processes because it breaks them down into smaller chunks to look at each area as an entity and then how the whole links together. The visual tools here are particularly helpful for taking a complex process and making it easier to see how it works as a whole (see Figure 5.9). It makes it easy to see where the wastes and challenges are to the efficient and smooth flow desired. The map is an overall view that makes it possible to see where to put further effort in a more detailed drill down so that the efforts going forward are directed in the right places.

Our First Vertical Visual Stream Mapping in Action

As we worked on this pictorial display we identified those areas for more detailed work and put into place plans for conducting several RIEs, which involved several exciting developments. For example, rapid stabilization units (RSUs) were planned. This

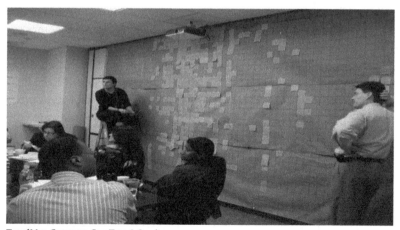

Top of Map: Customers, Core Team & Suppliers
Middle of Map: Tasks aligned to Process Owners & Project Milestones spanning 12 months
Bottom of Map: Identifies project completion end date, defination of reviews, freeze points & project name

Figure 5.8 Teamwork and the VVSM.

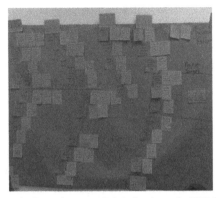

VVSM Solution Action Plan was derived from assessing gaps within the 7 critical clinical areas of care:

- Assessment
- Medical Nursing
- Medication Management
- Discharge Planning
- Treatment Planning
- Behavioral Management
- Environment of Care

Dark tabs are the WHATS? & Light tabs are the HOWS?

Figure 5.9 Reverse fishbone tool used to analyze gaps in vertical value stream mapping.

entailed designating specific psychiatric inpatient units as RSUs for patients, based on CPEP evaluations, who were likely to have shorter stays in the inpatient service; thus, those who could be rapidly stabilized and returned safely to the community for after-care. These units also doubled as "pilot" units where new standards of work would be implemented first until they were fine-tuned and mastered by staff, after which they would be rolled out to the remaining units in the hospital. This entailed developing standard work and then modifying it as any unanticipated glitches were identified and worked out so that the most recent standard of work reflected the best process to date if followed faithfully. Changes were presented to the steering committee for vetting and approval to ensure overall alignment with the department's true north metrics. The VVSM allowed for the first steps of looking at the entire continuum of care but on a small and manageable scale. Integration of services emerged as another priority from the VVSM and an RIE was planned that focused on improving the coordination of admissions processes from the CPEP to the inpatient service. This aimed at closing the symbolic distance between these two services by removing wasteful steps and providing a more integrated experience for the patients and less rework for the staff. Forms were developed jointly by the CPEP and inpatient staff that would capture information that could be built on rather than starting from the beginning and collecting the same information again once the patient reached the inpatient unit. These forms became dynamic rather than static documents.

Development of a Behavioral Health Support Team

A program development of note following our first VVSM was the creation of a Behavioral Support Team (BST). This was included in the provisions of the DOJ that required a reduction in restrictive interventions (use of restraints, seclusion, or 1:1 observation) and a focus on improving preventive strategies (e.g., recognizing the earliest beginnings of escalation or decompensation and intervening early before a crisis occurred). The BST comprised specially trained psychologists and behavior analysts who became our consulting experts in recognizing triggers to maladaptive behavior and who assisted teams with the development of plans to assist the patient and staff to recognize this early and to take more constructive actions. The BST consultative team was designed to assist treatment teams in the management of the most challenging behaviors utilizing positive behavioral support plans. The success of this program spread rapidly creating easy buy-in from the most dubious staff, psychiatrists among them. These plans were quickly and successfully reimplemented whenever a patient was later readmitted, again reducing waste of time, rework, and potentially negative outcomes.

Moving Beyond Acute Services

By January 2010, we were ready to move beyond the acute services of CPEP and inpatient units to our outpatient clinics. Our clinics were the next logical area to focus on and the adult outpatient clinic was selected to take advantage of New York State's recent announcement to revamp the payment structure for services delivered in such settings. In addition to our having to follow new regulations and regulatory survey processes announced by the State Office of Mental Health, fiscal opportunities involving the ability to bill for more than one service during a visit, required clinics to evolve to meet these new requirements and to take advantage of these reimbursement opportunities, especially as inpatient reimbursement was being cut. Lean processes enabled us to be well positioned and poised to succeed in this new environment. You will read more about the OPD redesign, an exciting venture in and of itself, in Chapter 8 of this book, which demonstrates how lean helped reduce caseloads while increasing capacity and total revenues.

Our Second Vertical Visual Stream Mapping

The Behavioral Health steering committee developed an increasingly sophisticated understanding of visioning processes as we ourselves matured and continued on our learning curve, a process we continue in earnest. We were more able to see beyond DOJ and oversight and more aware of the steps necessary to provide safety and quality care. Gaps continued to be identified and solutions sought. We became accustomed to finding more gaps as we successfully resolved earlier ones.

Our learning was supported by a new sensei that had been brought on board to work with KCHC as three other value streams within the hospital were identified: the general emergency room, surgery, and primary care. Sophistication in this sense, as is often the case, is a very relative term. We learned a great deal but have so much more to learn, but as our sensei coached us, that is what continuous incremental improvement is all about. Each visioning event in Behavioral Health represented an evolution from where we had been to where we wanted to go on our journey, and each step along the way allowed for the application of lean principles to hone our understanding of what steps were needed to move forward, constantly removing waste while striving to improve overall quality of care and increasing staff buy-in and participation along the way. Our understanding of true north metrics and the need for data to guide our decision making became clearer and clearer as the results of many, if not all, events were concretely realized.

Once the DOJ and plaintiff settlement agreements were signed, a new chapter was begun in the KCHC Behavioral Health story. In 2010 our next visioning event was specifically about DOJ. How were we going to achieve substantial compliance in all the areas, on each of the provisions, which were reflected on 300+ single-spaced pages of documents? The solution approach to this question was to once again utilize a VVSM approach for complex processes, the lean tool used to generate a project plan to allow activities within a value stream to flow without waste and to review the linked series of processes that occur throughout the value stream to organize the massive undertaking that would be required to respond to the provision of the settlement agreements.

During this VVSM event, the wall of a large conference room was covered in brown paper and the several areas of the DOJ provisions labeled on large white sheets of paper taped on top. This may not sound high tech, but it is very effective in encouraging all participants to "get their hands dirty" by taking part actively, writing on the wall, or drawing what the processes were or should be in the future. This fosters buy in by the line staff who immediately see the effect of their suggestions helping to make the changes, first on the wall and then in the actual processes at the worksite. One of our first collective thoughts was, "I don't know how we could do this without lean." There was so much that needed to be done, and of such import and with such scrutiny, that the organizing nature of the VVSM was an excellent fit.

Operation Flagship

As the days of this visioning event progressed, it began to take shape that this *was* doable after all; fear and frustration turned into excitement and hope. The techniques included looking at each of the numerous DOJ provisions separately and recording various activities under them that would aid us in fulfilling those provisions. Visual management tools—including using post-it's to represent the activities and placing them under the identified focus area, helped to make the tasks more understandable and manageable and permitted us to easily move items around the wall ending up with where they made the most sense overall. Accountable parties and teams for each area were identified, always including line staff, and enlisted. Their tasks were easy to understand using this approach. This led to greatly improved coordination and planning, which allowed us to tackle each of the areas for improvement, identify process owners for each area, establish appropriate metrics, necessary training, monitoring mechanisms, and timelines. We dubbed this stage of our evolution "Operation Flagship," as we hoped that this work would result in model programs that could guide and support other behavioral health facilities. It also seemed the perfect antonym for what one New York tabloid called us earlier, "a snake pit." Key safety and quality metrics were identified for tracking and included: reportable adverse clinical incidents, restrictive interventions (including restraint usage and 1:1 orders; we did not include seclusion as we did not use seclusion at KCHC), IM medications, recidivism (15 readmissions), and denials (refusal to pay for care by third parties).

A number of important approaches that developed out of this visioning event included the decision that we needed many more RIEs to achieve what was before us than is typical for an organization. In fact, we wanted twice as many. This necessitated additional lean support and two facilitators were identified for Behavioral Health to support our conducting one to two RIEs each month over the next year. Training about lean as well as the outcomes produced by the many events was also identified as essential and needed to be applied system-wide across Behavioral Health to attain and sustain the goal metrics and the overall outcome of substantial compliance with the substantive provisions of the DOJ.

In addition to RIEs, recall that lean also employs other techniques including JDIs and projects. The JDIs are those tasks that can quickly and easily be resolved. For example, needing a printer at the front desk to avoid wasteful steps is a JDI. A project is something more complicated and requires several weeks to months to achieve. An example of a project would be reducing overall length of stay for the adult inpatient psychiatric service. The use of lean projects was extensively employed during this year. Projects differ from RIEs in that whereas an RIE is completed in 4.5 days, projects can go on for months. These projects became the workgroups for the several key areas that the VVSM identified as necessary to meet the targets of the DOJ. The project workgroups each had a process owner and team leader assigned to them and representation from middle management and line staff, just like an RIE would. The process of empowering middle management and engaging line staff in decision making was both recommended to us by the DOJ subject-matter experts as well as thought essential during the VVSM to achieve the staff buy-in needed for attaining the compliance sought. In addition to approximately 14 RIEs, 13 workgroup projects and one data shop project were created out of the VVSM to achieve the transformation necessary to comply with the settlement agreements previously described.

Although fired up by the VVSM, this was a very exhausting year. Tremendous progress was made, but the staff did get a bit burnt out and subsequent visioning took this quite seriously. Although few organizations are faced with the type of burning platform we were at KCHC BHS, the possibilities of what can be achieved utilizing lean is striking regardless of how "hot" your burning platform is. The problem of burn out was identified as a gap and we recently dealt with it by forming a support group for staff as well as opened a "healing room" where staff could go and unwind when stress levels got too high. This room was equipped with a massage chair, soft lighting, calming colors and rugs, and the sound of a gentle waterfall along with aromatherapy and sensory modulation equipment.

Happily, our metrics reflected notable improvements, and the DOJ and other oversight agencies remarked on our continued improvements, while always reminding us that more needed to be done. We were on our way of working to achieving our goals when it became clear to us that our chosen target state (i.e., substantial compliance with DOJ mandates) needed to be modified: the goal shouldn't be "compliance"; true culture change wasn't about reactive mandated compliance. Staff wouldn't sustain certain processes because an oversight agency said they had to; staff needed to believe in what they were doing; they needed to own the process being created as they helped to create it, to be psychologically empowered.

Our next VSA—our fourth "pass" (value stream level reviews are conducted periodically realigning vision and metrics) for Behavioral Health in 2011—was a true turning point. Although the platform was still burning, it had changed into something no longer out of control, but manageable. Our goal was no longer about achieving compliance—for DOJ or any oversight agency (we continue to do excellently in state quality and compliance audits)—it was about achieving excellence. "Excellence Beyond Compliance" became the mantra, the overall Vision for 2011. Rather than our goal being to reach compliance, our goal would be to provide clinical excellence. Compliance would be a byproduct—a necessary byproduct, but a byproduct nonetheless. The requirements of the DOJ were actually quite in alignment with this. We realized that this is what the DOJ subject matter experts were trying to tell us all along.

Our visioning continues at the time of this writing with the theme of "Wellness, Recovery & Community Integration." Wellness, recovery, and community integration, although still a challenge for us, represents an evolution of earlier visions of patient-centered care, but now with the removal of the many silos created (each one

---

Lessons Learned

Conceptualizing the transformation as an internal process (to achieve excellence) as opposed to an external process (to achieve compliance) is an excellent example of an "insight" or "lesson learned" recorded in Box 9 of our A3, which you will read more about at the end of this chapter.

striving for excellence) and with their integration across the different services in Behavioral Health with the endpoint being the delivery of services based upon best practices within the overarching philosophy of patient centered, recovery-oriented care. Interestingly, during the previous DOJ visit, an expert commented that we had "developed cylinders of excellence." Our focus on integration, wellness, and recovery also incorporated medical services for behavioral health patients as well as successful and sustained reintegration back into the community. The most recent DOJ review noted, "the silos are gone."

Rapid Experiments

On a macro scale, the experience of KCHC in working to attain significant culture, process, and content change across the continuum of care in relatively short order serves as a "rapid" experiment for others looking to transform their institutions in radical and dramatic ways.

Lean provides the methodology, through events (RIEs and visioning), projects, metrics, and monitoring, but performance improvement is ultimately driven by the vision of the organization and the engagement and alignment of its staff with that vision. Gathering and using data and visual management tools and establishing standard work in this manner were new approaches for behavioral health and, in essence, rapid experiments in themselves. The visioning events are a vitally important part of the lean approach and the nexus around which the transformation continues to occur. Some of the initiatives you will read about in other chapters were designed as pilot projects, and other initiatives began in immature stages and then evolved with time as the process unfolded and other changes became apparent.

Performance improvement is a necessary part of the management of any behavioral health setting, and we found it profoundly useful in responding to regulatory and oversight agencies, regulatory requirements and mandates, as well as business planning. It provides a natural means for ensuring the use of best practices, with the tools to encourage inclusion and participation of all levels of staff, as well as those

---

Lessons Learned

This experimentation with the tools and techniques of lean was an important part of our learning curve. As we moved forward, and incorporated more lean tools into our solution approaches and management style, we had an "Aha" moment when we came to realize that in terms of performance improvement, lean was not an add-on but was, in fact, our departmental approach to overall performance improvement. It was not an addition to the quality management work we were doing, but instead was the quality management work itself.

we serve. It is data driven and, as such, provides a means for describing improvements in ways that are easy to understand and provides strong evidence for the improvements occurring in the organization. And it is not separate from lean, but one in the same. The Joint Commission, in its recent survey, commented that we were a performance improvement-driven hospital and that they were delighted to be taking away so many best practices from our facility.

The Completion Plans and Confirmed State

As we have learned in our lean journey thus far, continuous improvement is both our goal and our challenge. In particular areas previously identified as projects, RIEs, or JDIs may have been "completed" that is targets met; however, BHS as a value stream is in its fourth year, and a complete transformation will most likely take about 10 years for radical changes in both practice and culture to become the new norm for doing things. Why is culture so hard to change? This question is nicely tackled by Mann in *Creating a Lean Culture—Tools to Sustain Lean Conversions*.[8] Mann defines culture in a work organization as the sum of its individuals' work habits, and he has noted that "work related habits are just as difficult to change as personal habits." The behavioral science concept of "extinguish" captures this when talking about changing habits rather than the typical phrases of breaking or kicking a habit; to extinguish "implies a process, something that occurs gradually over time rather than an event producing a suddenly changed state."

What we would like to share with you here is what we consider to be "green versus red" in the lean lexicon for those areas in which we are reaching goals and those where we are not. In the spirit of making our journey visual and transparent, we will highlight here what has significantly changed and been sustained, as well as those areas where we are struggling and that need more focused effort to realize our goals.

Taking the broad view from 2008 to 2012 and looking over our yearly VSA Box 8 (Completion Plan) metrics, there are several major thresholds that have made considerable progress. We will take you through these areas and then follow with areas that we struggle with in terms of reaching targets.

PHYSICAL PLANT MOVE

The move from the G to R buildings had its nerve-wracking days but was very successful overall. Patients were moved from the CPEP and 10 inpatient units with considerable ease. Staffs were well informed, were on the same page, and functioned in ways planned to ensure the safety of our patients while not losing the new focus on quality of care we had come to expect of ourselves. There were numerous problems with IT and electronic failures in the new building that threatened a safe transition immediately following the move. The staff and leadership used our new

A3 thinking and built a "war room" in a central staffing area to detail and triage the mounting IT and facility issues. At one point our room was covered with 20- x 30-inch posters that literally wallpapered the room with items in need of attention. This was daunting but huddles every 3 hours with administration and various representatives from the physical plant department allowed middle and upper management to address each poster on a one by one basis while staff focused on delivering care to our patients.

Prior to using lean thinking, leadership may not have thought to make these issues visual in this manner or taken such an active stance to solve these problems. Earlier behavior would have involved numerous e-mails and conference room arguments; process not explored and persons blamed. This was a sign of leadership: staff and suppliers working in a new way utilizing A3 thinking.

STAFFING

An optimal staffing model had become considerably more established in CPEP and throughout middle management at this point, and we no longer had critical holes in our staffing pattern. In fact, compared to other hospital systems we were considered richly staffed. Clinical teams and infrastructure were formed with the addition of unit chiefs, head nurses, nurse managers, and local administration as well as the addition of psychologists, peer counselors, and a reinvigorated therapeutic rehabilitation division. Using historical data to determine staffing patterns that would meet patient demand was critical to ensure that standard work could be followed in any given area.

Importantly, in addition to the traditional clinical teams that were operating, specialized teams were developed to address specific critical areas of concern. Some examples of these included the developmentally delayed response team (MRDD) to assist the CPEP and inpatient services with the expertise and support necessary to better inform and manage care of this unique and challenging population that was not optimally served by our previous model of care or, in fact, by the larger city and state agencies. A BST grew out of the early success of the MRDD team and spread throughout the service to address particularly difficult to engage patients that scored high on risk assessments for aggressive, sexualized, or self-injurious behavior.

Building on this specialized "roving consultation team" model that supported clinical care teams, a readmission team under the leadership of a readmission review coordinator (RARC) was developed to address our readmission rates to both CPEP and inpatient services, which were both greater than comparable hospitals. With our new electronic record in both the CPEP and inpatient services, we were now able to track and trend these patients with reliable data to help us drill down to uncover root causes for problems as they occurred. The details of these analyses have helped us track and trend information by inpatient unit, clinician, and diagnosis, so that we could identify and tackle gaps uncovered in these treatment failures and build new and improved plans for these and future patients.

The data shop team was a major addition to our department. Numerous chart reviewers, data analysts, and IT specialists were brought in to ensure a more robust quality management department and to build better reporting mechanisms to inform leaderships and staff alike. Here we used consultants; eventually hiring a few to remain on staff to ensure that our clinical staff had a team on hand to work closely with their data needs. A number of practical and very helpful dashboards have resulted.

SILO APPROACH

A silo approach to care among the CPEP, the inpatient and the outpatient divisions, and our hospital's main medical ER continues, but overall integration between these key services has significantly improved from where they once were just a few years ago. The more we utilize A3 thinking to better understand who the various suppliers are and what their inputs are into any given process, the more we improve overall systems and increase the coordination of our work eliminating wasteful rework. The "us versus them" conversations are still there, but their frequency has greatly diminished. Using the patients' experiences and the input from our peer counselors as our guide to solving thorny problems has helped this transition. Although full integration remains a challenge, this will remain a major focus for us in the years to come.

Our greatest driver in breaking down these silos is placing team members from the silos on an RIE team for 1 week. It is almost impossible to come away from working intensively on a problem for 1 week without a better understanding of what the "other" does and why. More effective teamwork is typically the outcome with the likelihood of joint problem solving greatly enhanced.

Lessons Learned

The inpatient staff believed that "the CPEP did not care enough about sending patients up to the inpatient service with the correct medications." In an RIE exploring our admissions processes, staff realized the cumbersome and faulty process currently used for discharging patients from the CPEP and admitting them to an inpatient unit. Some of these defects resulted in some medications not following their patients to the floor. The conversation turned from finger pointing to collaboration in solving this dangerous problem within minutes of viewing all the steps of the process on a map. Again, the importance of visualizing process, a lean mainstay, proved invaluable.

COMPREHENSIVE PSYCHIATRIC EMERGENCY PROGRAM—
INPATIENT—OUTPATIENT DEPARTMENTS

As you can probably tell by now, the CPEP received the most focused activity early on at KCHC and is the most transformed service of our department. It is gratifying that many agencies have commented on the success story of our CPEP, and many come to study it in the hopes of replicating some of our processes. The inpatient service has also changed. Critical to the improvement of our inpatient services was the need for a better trained attending MD staff. Turnover in this division has been a problem, as several MDs left for "personal" reasons. It is our sense that many could not keep up with the pressures a rapid transformation required; others simply didn't have the ability or desire. We knew we would lose a number of staff, MDs included, and recognized that to move forward this would be necessary. The problem was that the timing of an MDs leaving was usually not optimal, and when several left within a short period of time, recruitment was quite challenging, requiring us to cover by moving staff from other parts of our department. Nevertheless, we were able to do this safely while successful recruitment of a new clinical staff was undertaken, with many hired and oriented to our department.

Fortunately, we are now in a position where we are being sought out by graduating residents and fellows who have either seen first-hand or heard about the transformation taking place at Kings County and deciding they wanted to be a part of that energetic evolution.

DATA

Of all that has changed at KCHC, this may be the most significant change of all. We were so data poor back in 2008, it was truly impossible to determine root causes of problems. When we did not have data, many solutions were designed for "symptoms of problems" and therefore those efforts were not successful. It was a "buckshot" solution approach hoping that something would hit the mark. Today, we are able to drill down into an area of difficulty and determine several contributing factors that enable a more scientific approach to the selection of a particular area of focus with the ability to also measure success after change was implemented. Our goal over the next few years is to use our data analytics shop to our fullest advantage. We are still learning how to use the data we are gathering most effectively but most probably are not yet using all the data we have to our fullest advantage.

We have, however, stopped "chasing normal variation" thanks to the use of control charts in our analyses. We are still data rich but information poor in some areas, and this remains a work in progress. Extremely helpful in this regard was the availability of consultants who assisted in formulating the right questions to ask to obtain the data needed and how to then analyze that data, thereby turning it into useful information for leadership and staff. Such consultants may be available to you by reaching out to your medical school or local college or university.

LEADING LEAN

Leading the lean journey for us has required a steep learning curve given our unique situation. Lean infrastructure has been put in place including a VSA once a year; project planning using the VVSM; regular process owners and executive sponsor meetings to guide our overall transformation, the oversight and input of the lean BH steering committee; and enterprise alignment by the full hospital's executive lean steering committee.

A continuous challenge is to move from top-down leadership with a reactive management approach to an organization that sees our line staff as problem solvers and stakeholders that can drive process change and incremental improvement from the grassroots bottom up. We continue to strive to become a true lean organization where there is respect, trust, collaboration, and team building between line staff and the various layers of departmental and hospital leadership. This remains a work in progress.

We have moved from a complacent and crisis-driven management style to a proactive approach but still have a great deal to learn about using the power of an empowered staff with a leadership team that is setting a vision together with those working in the trenches.

Our "green" successful milestones are exciting to share and celebrate with staff. Although it is always easier to discuss areas of accomplishment than our "red" areas, focused activity where we have not reached self-imposed targets and/ or not sustained efforts is vitally important to overall success (see Table 5.4). Sharing our areas of struggle is very important as we recognize that change is hard to achieve and even harder to sustain. There are three main areas that stand out as "red" and in need of further exploration and experimentation. These will be briefly reviewed next.

LENGTH OF STAY/RESTRAINTS

Length of stay (LOS) and restraint use have not consistently met their targets in either the CPEP or the adult inpatient services. There has been a radical reduction of 1:1 use; emergency medication (IMs and STAT meds) administration, and use of restraints, our target goals in these areas, are more recently being met.

We have just begun exploring key areas of treatment planning and getting data (e.g., seasonal, doctor specific and unit trends) to help areas in need of improvement. One project group that asked to work on this came up with a surprising finding that is worth noting. In the privacy of an interdisciplinary team approach to tackling LOS issues, a psychiatrist and nurse stated, "Well, we are working on so much that length of stay has fallen way down the list of things we are concerned about." This was very honest feedback and gave great insight to those trying to help in this area. If we are not focusing on something in a meaningful way, then it won't change. How do you work on team building, documentation, conducting therapeutic groups,

Table 5.4 Visual Management of VSA Metrics: Goal Met Goal *not me*

Metric	Baseline (9 units total)	Target (7W & 4W)	60 DAY (7W & 4W)	90 DAY (7W&4W)	120 DAY (7W & 4W)	150 DAY [7W & 4W]
Initial INPT High Risk Assessments within 8 hours	Adult Suicide = 98% Adult Violence = 98% Adult Sexual = 94% Child Suicide = 98% Child Violence = 13% Child Sexual = 87%	Adult = 95% Child = 95%	Adult Suicide = 100% Violence = 100% Sexual = 97% *Child Suicide 80%* *Violence = 80%* Sexual = 100%	Suicide = 97% Violence = 100% Sexual = 100% Suicide = 100% Violence = 100% Sexual = 100%	Suicide = 100% Violence = 91% Sexual = 100% Suicide = 75% Violence = 83% Sexual = 92%	Suicide = 100% Violence = 100% Sexual = 97% Suicide = 100% Violence = 100% Sexual = 100%
Nursing Assessment within 8 hours	Adult = 76% Child = 89%	Adult = 85% Child = 95%	*Adult = 83%* Child = 100%	Adult = 100% Child = 100	Adult = 100% Child = 93%	Adult = 97% Child = 100%
Psychiatrist Assessment in 24 hours	Adult = 58% Child = 70%	Adult = 85% Child = 85%	*Adult = 66%* Child = 100%	Adult = 80% Child = 88%	Adult = 84% Child = 87%	Adult = 85% *Child = 83%*
Psycho social Assessment in 72 hours	Adult = 76% Child = 20%	Adult = 85% Child = 85%	*Adult = 83%* *Child = 20%*	Adult = 94% Child = 100%	Adult = 92% Child = 93%	*Adult = 81%* Child = 100%
Medical Assessment in 72 hours	Adult = retrieve Child = retrieve	Adult = 95% Child = 90%	*Adult = 86%* *Child = retrieve*	*Adult = 94.5%* *Child = 87.5%*	Adult = 96% Child = 100%	*Adult = 94%* *Child = 75%*
Total Incidents Q1	340 (113 per month = 12.5 per unit)	10% reduction (106 per month = 11 per unit)	Adult = 6 Child = 7	Adult = 7 Child = 5	Adult = 3 Child = 14	Adult = 8 *Child = 14*
Reportable Incidents Q1	11 3.6 per month =.40 per unit)	reduction (3 per month = .33 per unit)	Adult = Zero Child = Zero	Adult = Zero Child = 1	Adult = Zero Child = Zero	Adult = Zero Child = 1

Sample Quality and Safety Metrics.

reducing the number of 1:1s, and still remember to deal with LOS? When too many balls are in the air, at least one will be dropped.

It appears LOS and restraint use are not just practice issues but cultural issues as well in our institution and therefore will probably require repeated efforts to achieve and sustain our goals. Thus far in these two critical areas, we have "picked the low-lying fruit" and had some modest gains. To drive deeper and have change in both practice and culture, we must work closer with the larger hospital and city agencies to build in the necessary components to reach the goals our patients expect and deserve. Our fifth pass at our VSA further developed the potential root causes to these gaps to ensure that we move forward with further improvement in these areas. Significantly, our department's first Lotus Award for Excellence was given to one of our adolescent units for achieving several weeks of being restraint free. Also, new processes involving social work and medical leadership are resulting in the successful discharges of many long-stay patients. Remember, lean is about continued incremental improvement.

STAFF MORALE AND TURNOVER

Introducing lean to an organization may bring morale up for many staff who will appreciate that lean provides a place for their voice and ideas to be heard and an opportunity for them to be a partner in bringing about change. Due to the ever present DOJ reviews every 6 months, sometimes our plans of corrective action require too much change with unrealistic timeframes. Organizations often get exhausted in years three to five of a lean journey, and we are seeing that now at KCHC. Lean can be seen as an additional responsibility rather than a more efficient way of operating. It is leadership's role to convince staff with evidence to the contrary. As Wellman and colleagues have noted in *Leading the Lean Healthcare Journey*,[9] "[To] truly transform organizational culture to embrace continuous performance improvement, leaders must intentionally behave in ways that support the philosophy of focusing on the patient and family, engaging staff and physicians as partners, and taking a long-term view." They describe the most important leadership behaviors as:

Leadership presence
Knowledge
Leadership participation
Tenacity
Patience

Wellman, Hagan, and Jeffries have further noted that the kind of leadership competencies needed for successful lean transformation "are quite different than those required in a more traditional work setting...[and must]...be tailored to foster, model, and reward the new behaviors."[10]

To address staff morale and burnout, we proposed some solutions after analysis and the completion of a staff engagement project. Several interventions have resulted from this, including the opening of a "healing room" where staff can go for quiet time, a staff advisory council to meet regularly with leadership, and more direct leadership support on each of the units modeled after our executive nurse–MD teams. Further, we have learned how to be more disciplined and responsive to staff's needs in our execution of lean, although per lean, we can always do better. Discipline is demonstrated by preparing for events 3 months before the event and by ensuring that standard work is concise and taught and displayed in a user-friendly way to be a support to staff and not a burden. We have learned many ways of seeing waste and problem solving thus far. Our goals going forward are to build model cells in all areas and to demonstrate the critical elements of one-by-one flow, pull, standard work, 6S, and visual management.

Insights

At the end of each lean event, time is taken to elicit insights learned from all participants. This helps bring the event to a close by reflecting on what worked, what hindered, and what could be done differently and perhaps better next time. It is again an example of incremental improvement efforts inherent in lean. What follows are key insights gleaned from designing and implementing events at KCHC.

"Two events a month, plus POCA and other regulatory demands—very difficult to juggle."
"Still learning how to lead by lean and practice lean as the way we practice, manage and problem solve."
"Staff and leaders have begun agreeing on using Lean to effect change."
"VVSM, VSA, and RIEs have helped shape and articulate vision and areas of focused improvement through event activity (prep, execution, tracking and success and failures in sustaining)."
"The A3 is a treatment plan for your BHS system."
"Build model processes and units, then carefully and slowly spread."
"Ensure process improvement incorporates all five true north metrics for an even approach."
"Much can be learned from failures."
"Change in practice and culture of management and care is not easy."
"Success happens in fits and starts."
"Lean is so much more than efficiency it is a way to lead and effect change in systems."
"Understand lean leadership and how to work with a sensei."

Some Insights From the Behavioral Health Services Leadership

MORE ABOUT DATA

If you take away nothing else from us about how to begin your lean journey, we would highly recommend spending a great deal of your time developing your data infrastructure. If forced to choose the single-most important change in both our culture and practice at KCHC, it is that we push one another now to "speak with data." That does not mean that we have data for every step of our practice; however, we are constantly asking questions that inform other areas to be modified in the electronic chart or in select data reports. Increasingly, we are able to speak with data and not only the usual quarterly reports or even monthly reports, but real-time data that can demonstrate trends easily. The development of a data dashboard for our service is not new in other industries but is revolutionary in psychiatric care. Building a robust data machine with an associated real-time data dashboard is a huge undertaking. This was painful for us but our greatest driver.

All electronic charts and white boards are not equal (we have learned this the hard way). A poorly designed electronic chart is not going to be an improvement over the old paper chart. If you have designed a user-friendly electronic chart, it does not mean that you automatically have data. Clinicians and computer programmers must work very closely together and learn new languages in order to communicate effectively. For our organization and most likely yours, this is a deeply humbling yet rewarding experience. Many of us still marvel that in just 3 years we went from paper and hand calculations to electronic records with built-in data reports. To demonstrate the power of this, let us share an example. In the early days if we wanted to do time observations of nurses and psychiatrists performing triage, then it had to be done with a stopwatch and most likely a small sample size. Now we trend triage times for both nurses and physicians by tour, clinician, and even by season. Drilling down into this endless data, we can post daily, weekly, and monthly reports by clinician for supervision purposes and for a bit of healthy competition.

Using data in this way has radically changed the way we manage, work, and problem solve. If you are just beginning your lean journey, we cannot overstate the importance of using data to transform your organization. It will help you identify

---

Lessons Learned

Learn from us here: Data, people, leadership, and end-users must have significant face time with one another to achieve an effective and efficient "data shop" for your transformation, we hold a weekly meeting to ensure that this face time occurs regularly.

problems, set baselines, establish targets, understand gaps in performance, and measure ongoing sustainment.

RESPECT

The stress of changing how we think about improving the delivery of care to our patients has often been overshadowed by the constantly changing landscape of the business of health care. Regulatory requirements and billing demands to stay solvent keep us spinning and in a state of sometimes seemingly conflicting loyalties. Through the use of tools like the A3 and practicing numerous new methods of visual analysis such as the VSA or VVSMs, we have come to realize that we are at times less adept project managers than dreamers of solutions. Let's unpack that last statement a bit.

Discovering as a group that generally we are not the best project managers was a bit surprising at first. There were and remain staff that pride themselves on following through; however, our natural practice is to not methodically plan the roll out of a solution to a root cause. We still forget to have all of the players in the room when we define problems. We still jump to implement without adequate experimentation and or communication. We still solve for symptoms rather than root causes and often this runs the risk of blaming a person rather than a process for less than optimal results.

These tough insights make us reflect on our respect for our patients and one another. KCHC is not alone in these struggles. This section is entitled "respect" because not taking the time to truly understand a problem that is impacting our patients and staff is actually disrespectful to all involved. Rolling out "half-baked" conference room solutions is a burden to our staff and not consistent with the philosophy of lean. Regressing to the mean and losing ground because of poor sustainment is a waste of everyone's time—again, not consistent with the philosophy of lean. When we find ourselves falling back into these patterns we pick ourselves back up and try to follow our lean practices. What is consistent with this philosophy is incremental improvement following the identification and elimination of waste. This is our mantra and what helps us prevent repeating errors we have learned from and encourages us to push forward when less than ideal outcomes result from any of our events.

PATIENCE

Be patient with yourself, your colleagues, and your boss—process improvement is really tough and you are going to make many mistakes, but from each, valuable lessons result that aide in your forward motion toward successful transformation. Remember that transforming both culture and practice is incredibly difficult and moving forward will not be a linear path but more likely one resembling a saw tooth.

No matter how "hot" your burning platform may be, only your focused joint efforts will win the day. Reflecting back, if we had slowed down at times and focused on the critical few issues for any given period of time rather than letting anxiety push us to take on more than the system could handle, then we may have accomplished and sustained even more than we actually did, and we did accomplish and sustain a great deal. Being a scientist of change can be tedious at times, and many well-intentioned experiments do not result in expected outcomes. The practice of being patient and disciplined in the use of your newfound lean tools and methods promises to bring lasting change. Lasting change means culture change, a lean driving force.

Part of being patient is taking the time to have every level of staff and leadership together, with your suppliers and customers (i.e., patients) at the table, when defining current problems and target states. A well-defined and data-supported problem with a clearly articulated vision will ensure your plans are supported for success. Couple this with ongoing communication of countermeasures to make necessary corrections and celebration of successes will help you lead your team on the path to a culture of process improvement. All of these steps take time but must be done if you seek sustained changes, and we know you are or you wouldn't be reading this book!

In the following chapters we will take you on a more in-depth tour of our lean work in some key areas of our department.

Notes

1. http://www.courts.state.ny.us/ad3/mhls/index.html, accessed December 9, 2012.
2. Byrne, A. (2013) *The Lean Turnaround—How Business Leaders Use Lean Principles to Create Value and Transform Their Company (p. xiv)*. New York: McGraw-Hill.
3. Liker, JK & Convis, GL. (2012). *The Toyota Way to Lean Leadership—Achieving and Sustaining Excellence Through Leadership Development* (p. 150). New York: McGraw-Hill.
4. Ibid, p. 152.
5. *On the Mend—Revolutionizing Healthcare to Save Lives and Transform the Industry (2010)*. Toussaint, J., & Gerard, R. A., with Adams, E. (p. 90). Cambridge, MA: Lean Enterprise Institute.
6. Liker, J. K. & Convis, G. L. (2012). *The Toyota Way to Lean Leadership—Achieving and Sustaining Excellence Through Leadership Development*. New York: McGraw-Hill.
7. Koenigsaecker, G. (2013). *Leading the Lean Enterprise Transformation* (pp. 94–101). Boca Raton, FL: CRC Press.
8. Mann, D. (2010). *Creating a Lean Culture—Tools to Sustain Lean Conversions* (2nd ed.) (pp. 14–21). Boca Raton, FL: CRC Press.
9. Wellman, J., Hagan, P., & Jeffries, H. (2011). *Leading the Lean Healthcare Journey* (pp. 39–43). Boca Raton, FL: CRC Press.

6

Comprehensive Psychiatric
Emergency Program

KRISTEN BAUMANN, REGINE BRUNY-OLAWAIYE,

AND RICHARD FREEMAN

Comprehensive Psychiatric Emergency Program

Chapter 5 presented an overview of both the vision of Behavioral Health Services at Kings County Hospital Center (KCHC) and how a change management system was brought in to transform the entire continuum of care from the psychiatric emergency room through the outpatient service. This global look at how the plans were developed and then executed between 2008 and 2012 for the entire service. It establishes a review of 4 years of work and gives you the reader an important reflective summary of our work to date. Chapter 5 helps place the work of the Comprehensive Psychiatric Emergency Program (CPEP) in context, noting that this is where the lean journey began at KCHC. The focus of this chapter will be on attempts at change just prior to lean, the radical changes lean ushered in with a focus on the stabilization of our triage processes, and finally linkage to our other services as lean moved from the CPEP to the inpatient and then to outpatient services.

The CPEP at KCHC includes the psychiatric emergency room; a six bed Extended Observation Unit; a 24 bed Crisis Residence off campus and a Mobile Crisis Unit. The psychiatric emergency room is where we have spent the majority of our time using lean, since it acts as the entrance to all of these services and serves as the admitting department to six adult inpatient units, three child inpatient units, a substance dependence unit, and the crisis residence. The psychiatric ER of CPEP sees approximately 550 adults and 100 children per month. The CPEP demonstrates a relative maturity compared to the rest of the hospital in utilizing lean as it moves into its fourth year of applying lean thinking. CPEP staff and leadership operate in a more cohesive manner than some other areas of the hospital because the philosophy of lean has gradually become embedded into the fabric of

Table 6.1 **Lean Improvements to the ER**

Before	After
Average LOS => 24 hours	Average LOS = > 14 hours
Average Triage = 60 minutes	Average Triage = 16 minutes
Patient Property Claims = 15–20 per month	Patient Property Claims = 1 per month

its overall operations and practices. The group of people working in CPEP prior to lean's arrival had to overcome a highly-publicized tragedy together (the death of Ms. Esmin Green). The team was intensely focused on exploring and implementing the necessary changes to prevent such a tragedy rom ever happening again. There could not have been a more compelling reason for action to start our lean work.

It is important to compare and contrast attempts at rapid change without lean and then with the tools and philosophy of lean (see Table 6.1). Much has been said about our burning platform and current state in Chapter 5. Let us take you a bit deeper into the CPEP.

In the late spring of 2008, CPEP was given a new leadership structure to help manage the massive changes that needed to be implemented, following a lawsuit and subsequent federal investigation which helped bring to light the need for changes in the CPEP and the inpatient services. Changes included introducing the CPEP director and associate director roles to support the existing ADN, head RN, and medical director roles. The medical director and nursing leadership at the time were managing a less than optimally staffed psychiatric ER in a building not suited for the volume and complexity of the patients that required their attention. The CPEP at this time could best be described as a reactive system in a state of crisis. The staff and local leadership had adapted to managing care in an overcrowded psychiatric ER. Although a new behavioral health building was under construction, financial realities within the city system at that time negatively impacted improvement efforts.

All of these stresses meant that executive leadership was struggling to implement changes in the CPEP and additional management was needed there to help execute critical and rapid changes. Prior to lean being brought in later that year (November 2008), a number of innovations were being explored. First, a new electronic chart with White board technology was being developed. The electronic chart replaced the paper chart and the White board was like a miraculous billboard with real-time patient information for our staff in the chart room and on staff computer screens. Second, plans to replace the hospital police role with specially trained behavioral health associates (BHAs) were underway. The BHA model had been developed at a sister HHC facility, and this new way of engaging patients to ensure a safe and therapeutic environment was very exciting for both staff and patients. Third, peer counselors (former patients) were being added to the staff in the CPEP. Additionally, new risk assessment tools were being developed to guide the triage and assessment phases of care. Finally, we were opening our new off-site crisis residence to help decompress the volume in our very busy psychiatric ER. All of these elements were being tried first in the older "G" building CPEP prior to November 2008. The thinking was to implement these as quickly as possible and then bring the best practices to the new CPEP "R" building in February 2009 upon its opening.

Without a lean system for change in place, these early initiatives were all top-down ideas put in place in an urgent manner. Communication was not always optimal among staff, middle management, and executive leaders across tours. Thus our reason for action then became more than just the conditions discussed above and now included how to bring about change quickly to a fragile system in a complicated area of care delivery and in a safe and sustainable manner.

The new leadership put in place in CPEP in the spring of 2008 found the existing practices and need for changes daunting. We knew what executive leaders wanted to do but were confronted with a large gap between the ideal state and the actual functioning of the CPEP. There was no chart room to gather in with staff, or even a mailbox system to communicate with the fast-paced 24-hour staff. There was one clerk working 9 a.m. to 5 p.m. Monday through Friday assisting RNs and MDs for the Extended Observation Unit (EOU) and the CPEP proper. Mobile Crisis and Registration were better staffed, but MDs and RNs still wasted hours each day on basic clerical tasks. When we began building a chart room, property room, supply room, and child overflow area, it became clear that this area lacked some essential physical plant needs for running an efficient CPEP. With these challenges in hand, staff and new leadership set out to build basic systems and optimize use of the limited space.

An underutilized "prisoner" holding area for patients in the custody of the New York Police Department was converted into a chart room with chairs, table, and a paper mailbox system. Later, three computers were brought in to alleviate the significant shortage of offices for clinicians in the old space. A property and supply room was established, and an office was converted to function as a child overflow area. The old CPEP was configured in a "Y" shape, originally with limited ability to separate between adults, children, or between the 72-hour EOU patients. This led to safety concerns for these three different populations. Great effort was required by staff to keep these populations apart and safe.

Once a chart room was established, "huddles" were instituted to help facilitate communication throughout the day. The first morning and evening change of shift huddles were of greatest concern. Early on, there seemed to be no sense of urgency on the part of the staff regarding triage, assessment, or disposition. To assess the impact of this, a chart review tool was developed and a part-time chart reviewer assessed the completeness of charting, which was our main data source. We learned through the real-time chart reviews that clinical basics like per-shift vital signs recordings and progress notes were not always fully documented. Also, the regulatory requirements of 30-minute triage, 6-hour evaluation, and maximum 24-hour length of stay were exceeded for some patients on a daily basis.

Without an electronic medical record, CPEP staff members were literally running from room to room to find the paper chart throughout the day, an example of the kind of wasted movement that lean looks to eliminate. The new associate director of the CPEP stood in the hall one day and watched staff going from room to room looking for patients, the chart, and one another. We next hired four temporary agency staff to fill the critical clerical gaps and to assist with charting as well as to act as "flow navigators." The addition of these temporary staff allowed clinicians to focus more on their clinical duties and less on clerical functions while improvements were developed and implemented.

The lean concept of "flow" was not evident in the CPEP—it was just chaotic. There was little connection between a series of tasks during the acute evaluation process. The clerical temps were used to answer phones and move patients and their charts from clinician to clinician to reduce the burden on the clinical staff. Later these temps used the chart review tool as a data set to help gather information and to also move care along in real time, thereby facilitating flow. These temporary workers acted as the link between tasks and disciplines until better processes could be designed. Their role was not a complete solution but a rapid way to bring order to an environment operating in disorder.

Between May and September 2008 the KCH CPEP probably saw more change than it had in many years. Although progress was uneven, staffs were trying to get on board as everyone fully recognized the need for massive changes in short order. If life in CPEP felt stressful before the tragic death of Ms. Greene in June 2008, the stress hit a fever pitch between June 2008 and Feb 2009. Just as improved charting began to take shape, the new electronic chart was instituted; just as the temps' data started coming in by hand we switched to a new system of collecting data through the electronic White board and the new electronic medical record (EMR). But neither the whiteboard nor the EMR was functioning reliably. The functioning and coordination of the peer counselors and the BHA program had kinks daily, and meeting triage, assessment, and disposition timelines were constant challenges. We were making many changes but staff frequently asked what was the overall vision that was driving all this change; how long could they endure working in an environment with so many changes being rolled out simultaneously; and how many of the changes could be sustained?

By September 2008, length of stay (LOS) in the CPEP (24-hour maximum by state regulation) had come down from an average of 30 hours to 8 hours. Huddles were happening on a somewhat more regular basis but lacked focus, and the new electronic chart was helping to reduce the overall chaos of delivering care, but was not yet a reliable system. Triage processes, registration, and the associated Whiteboard technology remained mostly accurate; shorter LOS did not however equal improved safety or quality of care—gains were still more erratic than consistent. Staffs were exhausted and not knowing what each day would bring brought on fatigue within months. We successfully brought down LOS and began working within the legal timeframes but we still were not changing processes—it was soon apparent that this was not a sustainable solution.

In November 2008, the New York City Health and Hospitals Corporation (HHC) brought in lean to support the transformation of the CPEP at KCHC. Lean had been implemented at some of our sister hospitals, and it was clear that despite our best efforts we were still struggling to sustain our many efforts, and we had a massive move planned from our old hospital to a new building. Our lean coaches helped us take inventory of our efforts to date and set a road map for change over the next few months.

The first formal target state for the CPEP in November 2008 could be stated as "have CPEP function with consistency"—that is, ensure safety and quality measures were consistently met for triage and for psychiatric and medical evaluations. We wanted a safe and effective triage system and rapid assessment and disposition processes along with the necessary training of all staff to ensure sustainment of gains while continuing to improve our processes. Triage practices were still quite variable across shifts and there was not agreement on which evidence-based risk assessment tools were to be used for violence, suicide, and cognitive impairment during the triage and early assessment of patients. Further, there needed to be clear role definition, with specific duties assigned to enable accountability and reduce duplication of effort. All agreed that the old crisis-driven silo approach to care had to be stopped and replaced with a client-centered team approach to achieve optimal results. The new and improved CPEP would be like a well-oiled machine, with each staff understanding their role and having a clear part to play in ensuring a therapeutic and safe environment in which our patients could be cared for.

Over time the target state changed to include better integration of all CPEP services (emergency room, crisis residence, mobile crisis unit, and EOU). Also, we needed to improve critical linkages with our emergency medical service (EMS) partners, medical emergency department teams, psychiatric adult and child inpatient teams, as well as chemical dependency and outpatient care teams. We were now committed to becoming lean. What did that mean? The multiple leaders of CPEP over the past 4 years took the lean true north metrics to heart each time we re-established our targets. Recall that the true north metrics include human development (HD), quality and safety, access and timeliness, and growth and financial.

Much of our work to date had focused on the first three metrics in CPEP. The first metric, developing our staff and our new lean leadership style (HD) has resulted in a true transformation in our thinking. This meant engaging our staff so they would define the multiple problems they faced, set goals and targets to implement corrective measures, and own the new processes to both achieve and sustain success. This new way encouraged staff and leadership to learn together and from one another. The "leader" is there to remove barriers to progress and to ensure that staff have all the tools they need to do their job well each and every day. Each staff member is there as a stakeholder and problem solver involved in continuous quality improvement and waste elimination. Process improvement went from crisis management to a sort of team sport!

The second metric focused on ensuring patient and staff safety and delivering quality of care each and every time, for each and every patient. We committed to exploring the best practices in our field and analyzed why we were not using many of them previously. We asked ourselves, "What are the barriers getting in our way to delivering quality care in a safe environment each and every day?" Finally, we pledged to ensure better access to our services and to remove waste from our system so that we could provide services to our community in a more timely manner. Our most recent target state for CPEP could best be summarized as: We commit to the continuous development of our people and improvement of our processes for the wellness and recovery of our patients in the most cost-effective manner possible.

The main metrics that have driven quality, safety and timeliness in the CPEP can be viewed in our confirmed state (see Figures 6.1–6.4). We have tracked MD triage, RN triage, disposition time, and overall LOS since January 2009. Data prior to January 2009 was not reliable and therefore is not shown.

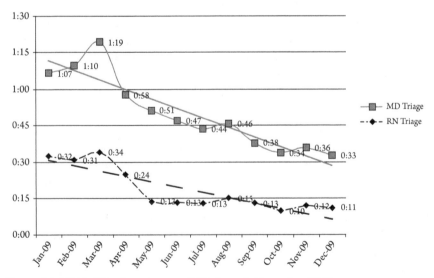

Figure 6.1 RN & MD triage, January 2009 through December 2009.

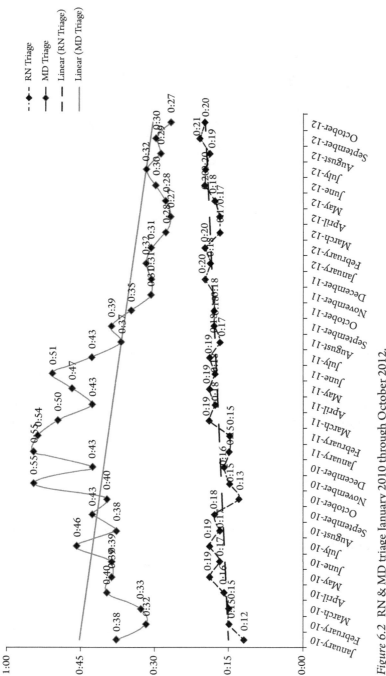

Figure 6.2 RN & MD triage January 2010 through October 2012.

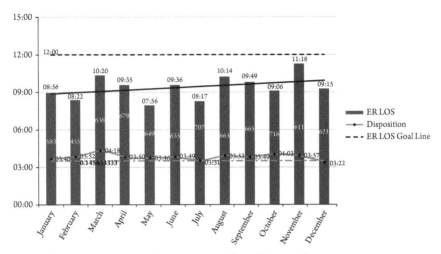

Figure 6.3 Disposition & LOS January 2009 through December 2009.

PART 1. Stabilize the Front End

One of the early "aha moments" we as a leadership team had was when we realized this "complicated A3 tool" our sensei was teaching us about was really just a structured treatment plan based on the scientific method! We realized we had never spent much time collecting data on our problems and certainly never explored root causes in a meaningful way. When we stopped and asked ourselves why no one had spent significant time studying problems in this way, everyone looked sheepish and responded that we never thought we had the time. Our sensei reassured us that this is common and was part of what we would work hard to undo. Root cause number one: there was no dependable, systematic way to address problems within the CPEP.

We started by looking at what had worked and what had not worked thus far. Some things did in fact work as discussed in our reason for action and current state (e.g., newly devised chart room, overflow room, use of temps). However, when we tried to bring about lasting change, we realized most things that we put in place worked for a while and then regressed back toward the mean. From April to November 2008 there were changes made, but the real gap was the lack of a system for change that would deliver results and sustain them over time. Our major tasks included transforming a fragile system with no standard work; no visual management; weak data systems; pushing versus pulling systems and the existence of silos between disciplines, to one in line with community standards. It was very difficult to undertake such a move when there was no model for a move of this scale for psychiatric patients that we could locate. How to take this recently retooled CPEP in

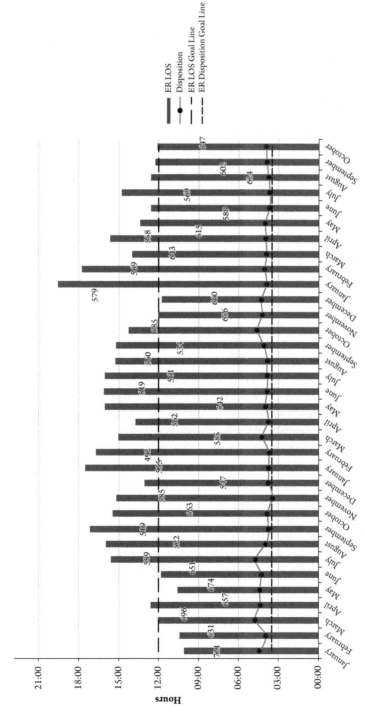

Figure 6.4 Disposition & LOS January 2010 through October 2012.

just months from its current 8000-square foot home to three areas spanning 16,000 square feet in the new building. Many did not want to leave this recently more stable CPEP as it meant rethinking everything because of a completely new layout and no more cross-utilization of staff. Staff and leaders had helped build a system that was beginning to be "functional" as compared to months earlier, and they were terrified of losing ground.

Lean thinking and coaches filled a significant gap in helping our executive leaders. Middle managers and staff got on the same page through the A3 process and with a vision of not just acceptable but superior care delivery and helped make the move from old to new hospital buildings happen without incident. Lean's coaching and structured system for changing both our business and clinical operations gave the team a sense that this new way of thinking could help us meet our next critical milestones. Staff that were exhausted and fearful began to perk up. The sense of learned helplessness lessened. The lean people sure had some strange ways of doing things—but really we needed help and what did we have to lose?

A major gap going into the new building was the lack of a clear triage and registration process; an effective search and storage of patient property system; and a reliable process for assigning our patients to a care team in the CPEP. To provide optimal care, these three key phases had to become as defect free as possible.

CPEP staff, leaders, and the executive team worked with our lean sensei for 6 weeks conducting one Value Stream Analysis and two Rapid Improvement Events to plan how to fix these issues by the day of the move. While keeping the "G" CPEP clinically in operation, we met in the new but empty CPEP for weeks planning for the new "R" CPEP. The architectural plans designed for the new CPEP were prepared years before and the then-designed processes did not always match what was needed now. Examples of this include one triage room planned when two were needed; no plans for a needed brief rapid treatment room; no overflow area for children; placing children in the adult EOB; huge areas dedicated for hours of waiting that were no longer needed; registration offices built in the back of the new CPEP; no clinical view of our ambulance entrance; and a space that was sprawling and difficult to directly observe and would therefore require more staff to safely cover it.

The newly formed lean BH Steering Committee, lean sensei, and CPEP leaders focused on building a series of connected processes ("cells" in lean terms) to assist in "pulling" patients through our system one by one with standard work detailing the steps from triage, search, and assignment to teams rather than the "pushing system" where patients at the end of the queue pushed those ahead of them forward. Pushing drove our system and is common in health care. Staff struggled with the concept of one-by-one flow, which refers to doing one thing at a time rather than batching tasks and patients, which in the end is more efficient and more patient-friendly. The concept of doing one thing well and to completion did not sit well with staff who were accustomed to (and prided themselves on) multitasking in the chaotic environment of a bustling inner-city psychiatric emergency room.

Let us unpack what has been said thus far. For the VSA we literally took a 20-foot by 4-foot piece of butcher block paper and mapped out with post-its (of different colors) the various tasks and disciplines involved from the moment a patient arrived at the CPEP door until they were discharged home or admitted to the six-bed extended observation unit (EOU), an inpatient unit, or transferred elsewhere. We then did time observations on the various steps depicted in the flow of the patient. Then we gathered 12 months of trended data on the various steps and also gathered data on staffing patterns related to the steps on the map. We gathered information from the laundry service we use as well as EMS and dietary services. We learned many things from our 4.5 days of working intensively together gathering data, making it visual, and discussing it together with our eyes on incremental overall improvement. For example, RNs were short-staffed during our busiest hours because they were completing their RN assessments in triage, which was causing a bottleneck in triage. (A great aha moment—so that was why triage took so long!)

Lean was teaching us to use visual management tools and time observations to assess staff workload patterns. When you map things out on paper rather than talk it out, people "see" what you are saying in a whole new way. It forces people to ask more questions, which leads to even more discoveries. The very act of writing forces us to listen to one another and focus on the problem rather than jumping to solutions. We had to learn how to set staffing patterns to meet our patients' care demands. For example, 11 a.m. to 7 p.m. was determined through data analysis to be our busiest hours; however, staffing was not scheduled that way. Lean was helping us use tools to better assess root causes of many of our problems so that our solutions could be optimized and tested prior to wide-scale implementation. Before lean we had one RN staffing pattern; after lean we had another that better matched patient need. Data was assisting in many ways.

We won't take you through every gap analysis, solution approach, and experiment but those of triage, search, property, registration, and assignment to team we think are worth sharing.

Triage and Technology

When we first began our work in the new "R" building CPEP the idea was to incorporate new technology such as Computers on Wheels (COWs) in the triage room to integrate some key elements. We had created a system whereby a patient enters CPEP's front door and was immediately seen by a team of clinicians and staff (MD, RN, clerk, and BHA), who did a quick visual triage. This was done to ensure safety by first doing a quick search and then whisking patients to triage where registration, triage proper, and securing of patient property would occur. We soon experienced problems with our design. Computers on Wheels were not reliable for the registration clerk, and there were too many people trying to work with the patient at the same time, leading to delays in the completion of triage. This approach also wasn't as patient friendly in practice as in theory.

TRIAGE IN STEPS

An RIE focused on coordinating triage and registration literally moved the registration clerk to the front door where a mini registration could be performed while nursing could begin a visual triage; then the BHAs could complete a safety search prior to the formal triage. We now had 1 x 1 flow of patients with pull, not push, between tasks! That is, each staff member could handle one patient at a time, completing their task, then handing off to the next staff member thereby not causing a bottleneck. Although there were a series of steps (patient had to move in this new set-up), each task had standard work with timeframes and triggers to pull to the next area. We finally could manage four major tasks with the majority of the patients and do so on average within 16 minutes (14 minutes less than the regulatory guidelines called for)!

Second Overflow Triage Room

The team developed a plan B for when four or more patients arrived at the same time to ensure we could continue to meet our triage demands. Plan B entailed calling overhead for a temporary second triage to be opened by another nurse to manage the overflow and then return to his/her duties once the surge subsided. We learned in RIEs that rapid experiments could show failures in ideas or highlight things that needed to be tweaked before being rolled out. Who has time to try things like this on the floor during the regular workday? RIE teams can with a well-defined problem and a structured approach and the protected time to conduct the analysis and rapid experiments. One huge advantage of this new design was that by having a mini- registration and a visual triage happen as soon as the patient entered the CPEP, the White board could be accurate and reflect real-time data on incoming patients. This helped the internist, psychiatrist, nurses, psychologists, and social workers and the rest of the team intervene quickly without needing a great deal of additional communication.

TEAM ASSIGNMENTS AND REGISTRATION

Our solutions and experiments were beginning to bear fruit—our gaps were becoming fewer. Each month we were getting closer and closer to our target metrics and the team was very excited and quite proud. By the way, lean emphasizes the importance of celebrating successes regularly. For years people had tried to tame the "triage beast." However, nothing goes without a few bumps, and we soon had issues with the White board accuracy because mini-registration clerks and back-end registration clerks would create duplicates in the system, assign patients to incorrect teams, etc. Executive leadership suggested, after much frustration, that perhaps this task was beyond the registration clerks in place and they might need to be removed from these duties. The team could then start from scratch with a new team utilizing the White board as a major visual management tool. Rather, one manager asked for, and was granted, 1 month to work in the registration area to get a better understanding of the challenges there. This is an example of going back to the first principle of lean; develop your people through understanding the problem by going to the Gemba. Within days it was apparent that the staff in this area had not been trained or retrained in many years in a structured and focused way. All training was currently being done by shadowing another clerk. Massive training went into effect for this area on all tours over 25 days and remedied the majority of the White board issues while satisfying the training needs of the clerks. This way of assessing a problem and addressing the root cause was new to us because of our lean training and A3 thinking. We were starting to see that with more planning and working with our staff, we could identify and address root causes of problems, and then the data-driven solutions would more likely be sustained.

The success of this series of RIEs related to triage took a few months and was a result of our A3 thinking. Prior to lean we did not consider the need for standard work and visual management. Ensuring work processes enabled staff to do one thing well and then to pull in the next task. Our thinking had been that we hire staff with particular licenses to do the work and that would be sufficient to achieve our goals. In our work exploring how to improve triage, we started to think about every aspect of what we did as needing to have five elements.

Figures 6.6 through 6.8 are all examples of lean visual management techniques.

Lessons Learned

Triage

1. **One-by-one flow**—Staff can really only do one thing well at a time so you need to set the system up to do that.
2. **Standard Work**—This is used to reinforce the new way of working developed in the RIE, use data to inform the staffing pattern. Standard work with the associated staffing pattern was the best way to lock in the improvement. Training your staff on this new standard and reinforcing it is the key to sustainment. If further improvements are made over time, update your standard of work and retrain your staff. Always date and post your standard work in the Gemba.
3. **Pull**—Create a way to **"pull"** staff and patients through (i.e., patient arrives and has a visual triage and mini registration, then moved quickly to a search for safety, then walked to triage, then BHA pulls patient to property area, then assessment completed by assigned care team).

(continued)

4. 6S—All the supplies needed are where you need them (called 6S). Nurses don't go running around for a syringe every time they want to draw blood, it is right there, where it should be, and in the same place in similar rooms. Much of the waste identified is the lack of planning for what we need, where we need it, for when we need it.

   - Sort—Distinguish between what is needed and not needed and remove the latter.
   - Stabilize—Enforce a place for everything and everything in its place.
   - Shine—Clean up the workplace and look for ways to keep it clean.
   - Standardize—Maintain and monitor adherence to the first three Ss.
   - Sustain—Follow the rules to keep the workplace 6S-right—"maintain the gain."
   - Safety—Eliminate hazards. (The sixth "S" helps maintain the focus on Safety within our Lean events and embed safe conditions into all our improvements.)

5 **Visual Management** Tools—=All these functions are supported with easy-to-read and understand visual aids to support the functions (i.e., labels on drawers, instructions, data on week's performance; see Figure 6.5).

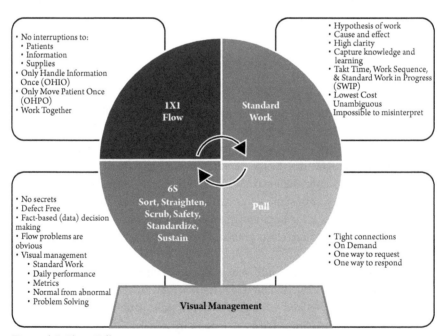

Figure 6.5 Flow Cell.

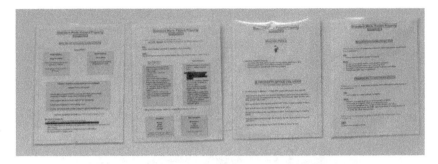

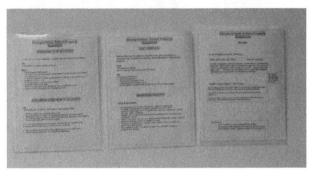

Figure 6.6 Standard Work.

Part 2. CPEP and BEYOND

As mentioned in Chapter 5 (page 145) a Vertical Value Stream Mapping event (VVSM) was held in August 2009 and again in March 2010, to use A-3 thinking). Vertical value stream mapping spelled out the direction and steps Behavioral Health would take over the next 12 to 18 months utilizing a project planning process. Although the focus was now spreading to other clinical areas, CPEP remained in the centerpiece of the department's upcoming process changes. The first event to begin the process of breaking down the barriers between CPEP and the inpatient service involved patient property. We wanted to start with something concrete but also something that was causing great angst to both services and most importantly to our patients.

PATIENT PROPERTY

Imagine that you are hospitalized. What are your expectations about the property you came to the hospital with? Would you be focusing on whether or not your property would be there for you upon discharge? Most probably not! That you would arrive with personal belongings and leave with those same belongings is simply taken for granted.

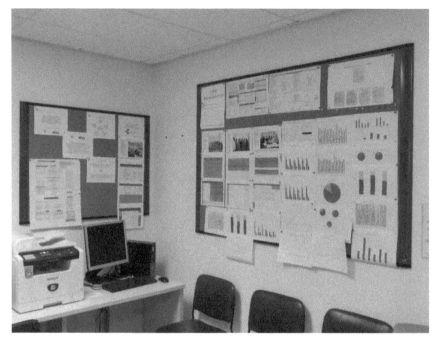

Figure 6.7 Chart room with DATA.

Prior to June 2009, however, this was not the case in the CPEP. Although there was a loosely defined process in place and patient's property was secured and logged, it could not always be accounted for upon discharge from either the CPEP or the Inpatient Service. Alternatively, there were often several packages left in the property room for individuals who were no longer patients in the hospital. This resulted in frequent patient complaints and claims to recoup money for lost property and much waste of staff time searching for lost property. This rapid improvement event had a straightforward confirmed state: patient claims for lost property set at zero.

During our preparatory work for this event, we found out that on average a claim for lost property took about 7 hours of staff time to investigate and report. Hospital police reported at that time that on average there were approximately 15 to 20 claims per month. At 7 hours per claim and 20 claims per month, the total staff time was 140 hours per month. There was significant potential for savings by eliminating wasted staff hours and without needing to reimburse for lost property. This RIE, like the one on triage times, has been sustained and has essentially eliminated missing or lost property in the CPEP and between the CPEP and the inpatient services. How was this done?

A major barrier and root cause to property left behind was discovered during the RIE. All property of value was picked up by the Property Office daily and secured.

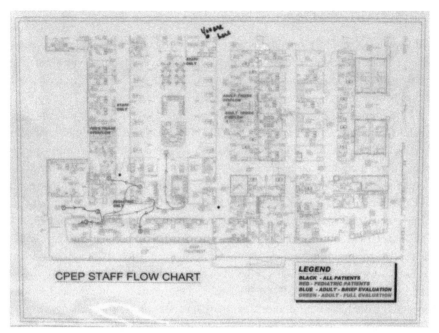

CPEP STAFF FLOW CHART

LEGEND
BLACK - ALL PATIENTS
RED - PEDIATRIC PATIENTS
BLUE - ADULT - BRIEF EVALUATION
GREEN - ADULT - FULL EVALUATION

Figure 6.8 Staff flow chart.

It could only be retrieved 9 a.m. to 5 p.m. Monday through Friday. If staff wanted access at other times, they would have to call an Administrator on Duty (AOD) to retrieve items or the patients had to come back during the Property Office operating hours. The team designed an entirely new system where pick-up was less frequent but valuable property was secured in a cabinet by hospital police just outside of CPEP due to the 24-hour operation of CPEP services. Further, there were strict protocols put in place for tagging, bagging, accountability of inventory, and organization of items in the property rooms on both services. Photos were posted in property rooms of how they were to be left and it was clear to all who entered if things were in place or not. Staff jumped at the chance to help bring about these changes. We had hospital police, AODs, property officer, peer counselor, and representatives from both CPEP and inpatient on this team. All were invested in fixing this issue as many hours of their days had been consumed with searching for items, calling various offices to gain access, and being on the receiving end of patients and their family members being frustrated and angry. As of October 2009 this is no longer a hot button issue because of stable processes with clear and posted standard work serving to maintain the gains achieved.

RAPID STABILIZATION UNITS

By October 2009, CPEP operations were better integrated (i.e., registration, triage, property and assessment); however, integration with the inpatient services remained problematic. Although confirmed state trends for both MD and RN triage, as well as disposition times, remained on target, LOS for CPEP was variable. "Pull" did not drive the admissions process. Rather, CPEP continued to "push" their patients on to the units. Although CPEP average LOS at that time was approximately 11 hours, the inpatient LOS could be as high as 32 days. The long inpatient LOS (resulting from many factors including our being a "safety net" hospital, homelessness, the undocumented legal status of many of our patients, to name a few) had a significant impact on CPEP's ability to maintain a consistently acceptable LOS. How did that translate to the end user? Basically it results in frustrated psychiatric patients and families, as well as the CPEP requiring diversion for ambulance calls to prevent overcrowding of the psychiatric emergency room, and therefore, our not being able to serve as many patients as we could otherwise. The goal of the rapid stabilization unit RIE was to establish standards of work that would subsequently affect workflow and process through the establishment of model, or pilot, inpatient units. These changes in turn would impact patient care by removing waste during the admissions and treatment processes and ensure continuous treatment to enable more rapid stabilization. This would translate into a shorter inpatient length of stay and an increased availability of beds to admit patients to and therefore not requiring us going on diversion as often. The target was for this model to then be spread to other units, ultimately helping the entire system and reducing the times the CPEP would be on ambulance diversion. The expectation was to reduce the inpatient LOS by half by treating and releasing patients within a 15-day period. Flow would be optimized and more patients would be served, hopefully with improved patient satisfaction.

There were high hopes that not only would this RIE address this real-time issue of bed availability but that it would result in a long-term paradigm shift in the minds and actions of treating providers. Rather than limiting treatment to traditional workday hours, the existence and success of the Rapid Stabilization Units (RSUs) would redefine and conceptualize patient-centered care as responsive to patient needs no matter when the need arose.

The plan put in place by the RIE recommended that the RSU team *come to* CPEP to meet the patient and *begin* inpatient treatment there. This process was expected to reduce patient anxiety by meeting some of the staff that would be treating them once admitted. It was also expected that this process would expedite admission to the floor. The impact of the RSUs would be significant for CPEP in that it allowed both entities to work synergistically by attempting to identify those patients who would be minimal users of service time and could be reintegrated into the community quicker.

Imagine CPEP and its multiple components as a four-lane highway. Some lanes are at a standstill and some are moving at about 5 to 10 miles per hour, but it is stop-and-go traffic. *When this RIE occurred and the pilot commenced, it was as if a previously bottlenecked lane opened up.* Even if its capacity was limited, there was constant "flow." That constant flow now translated into improved quality of care for those patients who were in that lane. Psychiatric treatment was initiated earlier; they were now less likely to be the subject of a psychiatric emergency, stat medication administration, or restraint secondary to frustration at delays in internal movement from CPEP to the unit. However we did run into some barriers, for example, it was difficult to get the teams to come down on a timely basis since they were busy treating patients on their unit. Although this ambitious RIE did not help reduce the total LOS in the CPEP, the individual RSUs themselves did have a reduced LOS for a period. The RSU concept, however, was not sustainable because of unintended consequences, including disruptions to the overall functioning of the inpatient service.

In February 2010, the RSU Pilot was revisited with a follow-up RIE. The purpose was to re-evaluate the restrictive criteria for admission to these new pilot units, as well as the requirement for RSU teams to come down to CPEP. With the population that KCHC serves, it was difficult to meet the criteria for the original RSU model. Additionally, the stress on the staff of the RSU became apparent and it was decided to continue to utilize the units as pilot units where new policies would be rolled out and perfected before being generalized throughout the hospital but to no longer keep the short-term nature of the units. There was also reconsideration of the requirement to have staff come down to initiate treatment in the CPEP. This enabled patients to be transferred to an inpatient unit faster. The RSU pilot was an interesting experiment but one that in the end did not succeed fully as planned and was reworked accordingly. (At this time, there are no longer pilot units, as all units have now adopted all policies. Also, new LOS reduction processes have been put into place which are taking hold and being effective.)

Exporting the new processes onto all the remaining units wasn't so simple. In our excitement to spread the initial successes we saw on the RSU-pilot units, we lost touch with some basic facts. RSU gains were made because the staffs on the units were intimately involved in resolving the identified problems, a basic lean principle. When the attempt was made to spread these new findings we found ourselves imposing a new way on units that had *not been* involved with the experiment stage. It appeared that we had reverted to a top-down approach that is not in keeping with the lean principles of respect for people and the process. This was a major lesson learned. Information sharing, training, and support during a transition phase from the old to the new standard of work is more likely to be sustainable.

REASSESSMENTS AND PRACTICE GUIDELINES

Although CPEP had shown marked improvement in performing initial assessments, as always, there was still room for further improvement. Diagnoses were not always made in a timely fashion, and there were a disproportionate number of patients who were given "diagnoses of exclusion" (NOS). Systemic issues also surfaced, as there was difficulty finding updated correct diagnostic options within the electronic medical record (e.g., ICD codes rather than DSM diagnoses were programmed into the EMR) and there was variance in the quality of work and documentation performed across disciplines. Rather than using evidenced-based treatment standards, treatment was guided by symptom presentation rather than underlying diagnoses. Treatment and aftercare plans were therefore also limited because of inadequate or incomplete diagnostic practices. The consequences of this current state were inadequate diagnosis of patients, treatment delays, increased length of stay, increased risk of the occurrence of untoward events, and waste of resources.

Staff routinely struggled to implement routine ongoing assessments. These were not seen as part of the assess–treat--reassess cycle of care; further, the overall process was not well documented. There was no real standard of work and considerable confusion about the who, when, and what aspects of the ongoing assessment process.

Over the course of the re-assessment and practice guidelines RIEs, there were several tools used and rapid experiments conducted these revealed suboptimal staffing levels as well as the need for clinical tools to aid the clinicians in making appropriate diagnoses and, accordingly, implementing the correct treatment plan. Let us take you through some of the gaps and solutions we came up with. The analysis of our takt time (defined as available time divided by patient demand) and bar charts of other data revealed the need for additional case worker staff to assist the licensed clinical staff so that they could meet the content and time requirements for quality patient evaluations and documentation Gaps were also uncovered in the utilization of floating attending psychiatrists, as opposed to doctors designated and wanting to work in the CPEP. The understaffing of caseworkers in the CPEP and use of "floaters" revealed elements of an earlier crisis-driven model of operation that made it difficult for staff to organize their work and negotiate priorities. Put simply, the licensed clinical staff could not meet the pace of demand for evaluations because they were too busy doing concrete service tasks more appropriate for caseworkers. These findings were discussed at the daily out-brief during the RIE and were followed up on after the event by the director of social work and director of CPEP.

Once staffing patterns and demands were better understood these events moved on to provide tools to help deliver the quality and safe care we had come to expect of ourselves. The development of evidence-based practice tools (see Figure 6.9 below) was helpful in guiding clinicians to arrive at accurate diagnoses and provide proper management for KCHC's top three diagnostic categories: schizophrenia, bipolar disorder, and major depressive disorder.

The information technology (IT) department was instrumental in adding drop-down menus to the EMR to facilitate the diagnostic support tools and treatment algorithms. We have found that IT fixes cannot be used for everything but can provide helpful prompts in a number of areas. In addition to EMR prompts, all our

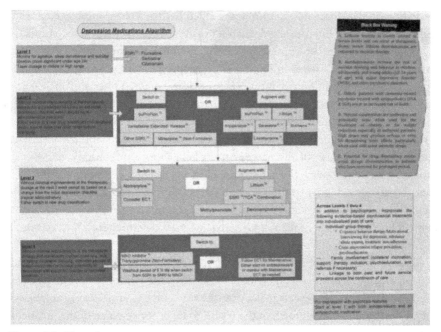

Figure 6.9 Algorithm.

treatment algorithms are posted in the unit chart rooms in keeping with the lean principles of visual management and standard work.

Rapid experiments were also conducted to test the feasibility of providing a structured template for documentation emphasizing consistency and thoroughness. Some highlights: the Subjective, Objective, Assessment and Plan (SOAP) note was developed; the Extended Observation Unit Treatment Plan was redeveloped; and the "Huddle" (frequent, crisp meetings to share clinical information) format was also designed and implemented. All of these products were generated to provide a framework of information needed in the electronic medical record or to aid in the daily verbal communication process. Experience has taught us that staff development remains a key issue when developing and introducing such new tools. After new products are introduced, there is a constant need to train, review, tweak, and support staff. If the support is not there even the best tools will be rejected and not help you reach your goals.

REPEAT ADMISSIONS REVIEW COMMITTEE

Before we take you through our data and final insights let us share with you our most recent adventure: trying to tackle readmissions back to the hospital shortly after discharge. KCHC had a higher rate for this than many of our sister hospitals.

An RIE created a whole new clinical team called RARC. This group is tasked with collecting, tracking, interpreting data about readmitted patients, and recommending plans of action for aftercare to prevent readmissions in the future. During the RIE preparatory work we found that there wasn't a standard of work, there was a lack of clear policies and procedures, a lack of clearly defined roles and an absence of data driven outcomes pertaining to discharge and readmission. The RARC RIE shaped and defined the process and was successful in establishing current practices for evaluating patients that return to the CPEP within 60 days and the inpatient service within 15 days of discharge. After establishing expectations, unit-based teams were able to review the gaps in previous treatment and aftercare plans that contributed to our higher readmission rates. It also broadened staffs' clinical assessments to incorporate the patient, family, and community voice. This led to changes in the follow-up treatment plans which now incorporate stronger support services to facilitate our patients' successful return to their community.

Through the efforts of RARC, readmission rates for CPEP dropped from 21% to 14% on average. This surpassed the initial goal set by the RIE of 18%. Data that has been collected thus far reveals that a primary reason for readmission is homelessness. Efforts are being put forth in the CPEP to incorporate some of the inpatient tools used by the RARC committee (i.e., the use of the monitoring, referral, and linkage unit staff), which help to track patients upon discharge for up to 90 days post-discharge. Additional in-depth discussion regarding the RARC on the inpatient unit will follow in Chapter 8 (page 234).

Insights

REFLECTIONS

The results of using lean to tackle some issues that had stymied leaders of the CPEP for years was impressive and very exciting because it worked in many different critical areas. Not every RIE or every element of an RIE worked, but overall one could look back over 6 to 12 months and see that things were dramatically improved and, equally important, sustained. For staff it was a welcome change to have an articulated vision with a system of implementation that worked and that they shared fully in. For middle managers, it was welcomed as a way to link staff with executive leadership. Using A3 thinking as a way to think and practice helped get everyone on the same page—literally. The method of focused problem solving on an 11" X 17A-3-piece of paper helped us reach consensus for thorny problems, plan in more meaningful ways, and design experiments that would lead to change that lasted. Working in this way was much more collaborative, focused, less exhausting, and more empowering.

As mentioned in our current state before implementing lean-led changes, we were able to identify problems and roll out solutions. Examples included the use of temps, converting offices to chart rooms or child overflow rooms, and so forth. The difference *with* lean is we were learning to plan and be thoughtful about which problems to go after—we are able to be less reactive and more proactive. This was the result of A3 thinking, staff-leadership collaboration, and executive level support. Our solutions began to solve root causes, not symptoms of other issues. Many of our previous solutions were not half bad considering there was minimal analysis, limited usable data, and suboptimal communication about the change! Most of our pre-lean solutions, however, failed to sustain because of one or all of these reasons. Far too often, we previously would roll out a major initiative by memo or a quick huddle with the day shift staff without input from the other staff.

After we began our lean journey, we received positive feedback from patients, families, and even EMS workers. Many noted how different the experience was and were impressed with the increased timeliness with which our "front door," the CPEP now operated. CPEP from April 2008 to March 2012 demonstrated what a group of people could accomplish when they were focused and clear about what needed to be done and were supportive of this effort. It was impressive for the team to work through root causes and roll out and sustain powerful solutions even with significant leadership and staff changes throughout this period of time. RIE teams and process owners worked evenings and weekends to perfect standard work and make videos to demonstrate the new methods they had worked so hard to create in an effort to teach others.

Much of what worked could best be described by using our "new compass" the True North metrics. First, we used our "experts"—our line staff (including our newly added team of peer counselors) to help articulate and solve problems. Staff appreciated being valued as stakeholders and problem solvers. They were encouraging one another to follow new standard work and coming up with solutions to barriers through newly devised standard of work. Second, with a focus on the patient's experience of quality and safety, staff could get back to what brought them into the field of behavioral health rather than engaging in turf wars and designing practices around their needs rather than the patients. Third, we learned access and timeliness does not always mean "working faster"—just efficiently and with clear purpose. Fourth, we learned that when we do focus on Human Development, Quality, and Safety and Access—we see more patients, which means greater opportunities for service to our community as well as revenue for the hospital. Here it is worth noting that we were seeing more patients as the overall LOS came down. We are now focusing on coding, billing, and helping patients to become insured, which will help our overall return on investment. The following chapter has more financial success to share pertaining to the outpatient department.

LESSONS LEARNED

An active "roll up your sleeves" approach to leadership works. If you want your staff to go down a tough dark road of unknowns, then you better lead by example. If you don't understand a process, then ask the staff in that area to teach you the job for a few days so you can better understand the problems. Go to the Gemba, and go often. Share any data you have with the staff regarding the process you are trying to change in real time and set aside time to discuss trends in data to work toward continuous improvement. Too often administrators redefine roles, jobs, and processes they do not truly understand or only look at data with other administrators without going to the actual worksite to see the context.

An example of how we work differently now is demonstrated by our triage times. To radically change both MD and RN triage times, we broke the data down by tours and then by names and worked with the individuals who were outliers. The RNs as a group came around quite quickly. Their outlier times generally had to do with a patient that was not voluntarily in the CPEP. The MDs for a time struggled with new protocols at time of triage. As we began posting weekly data with doctors names attached, subtle peer pressure helped get those numbers back on track.

Visuals, standard work, updates on dry erase boards, and frequent, structured huddles, and Gemba walks help manage defects in the process and provide opportunities for real-time problem solving. We used to train our staff by having the new member shadow someone else within their discipline. What we gained from this approach was that no two people were doing any task or process the same way. There was so much variation it made it nearly impossible to look at your current state of doing things from a qualitative or quantitative perspective as there was no one standard way. Now staff have standard work for critical steps in our processes to ensure we are doing things in a similar way (because it was shown by them to work) across tours and this is shared with new employees. Trends in data help to highlight any problems in our processes—not just variations by clinicians. Data, updates and huddles help reinforce our continuous learning and incremental daily improvement in quality.

The electronic chart and White board technology are remarkable, if not always perfect, tools. Prior daily data collection was done by hand and never gave you the depth of data upon which to build lasting solutions. The kind of data we could manually gather sometimes even contributed to a crisis-driven care delivery and management style because we were not always looking at data in context but being reactive to it. Too much of a good thing can also be a problem. We went from having virtually no data to drowning in data at one point! Lesson learned—keep data meaningful and relevant to the staff in that area and keep it simple. When we look back to the spring of 2008 when we had a paper chart and no efficient data-gathering and reporting system in place; we were truly operating in the dark. However, the electronic chart is not a panacea. We do not recommend rushing to build one. We wasted a great deal of time and money in a hastily built electronic chart that we are still trying to remedy. Lean teaches to sit with a problem and understand every facet before moving to a solution. We recommend that IT staff and clinicians use lean or a similar methodology to build yours.

Lean is a team sport. Team work, collaboration, and the deep problem solving required to make changes to both practice and culture in a chaotic place like a psychiatric emergency room doesn't just happen; it must be nurtured and facilitated. Lean is not something you implement or deploy; it is something you and your organization become over years. Don't focus on results—focus on improving processes that impact the quality and safety of the care your clinicians deliver and your patients receive. If you focus on processes you will develop things that can be tested, repeated and forever improved upon—things that can be sustained. Our triage system has gone through three cycles of improvement and is ready for its fourth. The reason it has been sustained for 3 years . . . we focused on the five core elements of a cell: 1 X 1; Standard Work; 6S (a lean tool of organizing the workspace so that you have what you need where you need it); Pull; & Visual Management. We developed interlocking cells that have triggers to pull to the next cell all supported by data and the right staffing patterns. Our data show we are ready for the next round of continuous improvement . . . and we are ready!

Staff Insights

1. What I remember most about my breakthrough experience is the excitement I felt in the pit of my stomach for my first event and each and every time I have been part of an event. The excitement resulted from the fact that I knew this "tool" called lean was POWERFUL! I see it as powerful for a few reasons. First, because lean is a *proven* method of sustainable change. Second, because it has been vetted and adopted as the method by which change will occur at KCHC . . . .in other words, the "head honchos" approve! It is no small feat to change corporate culture and to have leaders of a major health system change the way they think about how they will go about their daily operations (top down).

I also felt very proud. Proud to have been found worthy to participate. Proud because I felt trusted. I felt as if my supervisors and colleagues really saw value in my opinion and are willing to put their "daily work life" in my hands. Last but not least I felt a little trepidation, dread, and fear. Much like that feeling most medical students have that they are charlatans and it's only a matter of time before they are "found out." I have felt fearful that the 4.5-day time frame was not enough and that the task at hand was beyond my ability to solve. This feeling usually surfaced around "Tequila Tuesday" (as the challenging Tuesday of an RIE week is affectionately called) after report out. But then, as time moved forward, that fearfulness was gradually transformed by several aha! moments, after which a contented sense of calm comes over me as I realize the problem was never MINE to solve in the first place and that

(continued)

I needed to trust in the process. Then a different type of excitement would emerge. It is a kind of nervous excitement brought on in anticipation of the final report out.

Before my tenure at KCHC I have been part of several team projects. However, I have never had an experience quite like lean's RIE or VSA. Being an early career psychiatrist, I am in awe of my progression to a position of leadership and am in even more awe of the "behind the scenes" workings of how to actually go about running a hospital. I feel humbled and privileged by the opportunity to be exposed to so much so early on in my career. Lean has made me feel even hungrier to learn because it gives me a sense of security that no matter what problems arise, I will be able to reach out to my supervisors and peers and find a solution using the tools of lean to guide me.

The workplace has changed for the better. Staff feels more freedom to be vocal about things that require attention because they know it will be heard and there is a mechanism in place to address it, as opposed to being ignored and endlessly living with the problem. I am happy to have the opportunity to be both on the front lines AND to have the 30,000 foot view in the process. It gives me a 360 degree understanding of what the issues are and informs me in a way no other situation could.

2. I was a Nurse's aide when I worked in the G Building, I continued my studies and obtained my RN while still there. As such, my duties changed significantly when my role changed. What is most striking for me is the transformation from disorganization to organization lean helped bring about. Having a standard of work for such a large operation is invaluable. Our way of working is now completely different. Before lean there was limited engagement with our patients. There was overcrowding and little to no external support. There has been tremendous change from then 'til now. I must say that I was a skeptic at first. When I walked into my first RIE and I looked at the reason for action on the board and was told that the group was charged with developing a solution for the issue, I thought to myself, "It's not possible! It can't be fixed!" I am happy to say, however. that today, I am a convert. At the conclusion of the RIE I realized, "This can actually be done! And in 4.5 days!" I am impressed by both the components of the process and how it helps to inform the solutions proposed. Fresh eyes are a good example of this. I would have never realized just how vital an individual who is completely removed from the process would be and how integral he or she is in developing a workable solution that is sustainable.

7

Lean and Inpatient Psychiatry

ROUMEN N. NIKOLOV, AKINOLA ADEBISI, AND LINDA PARADISO

The face of inpatient psychiatry is changing very fast these days. All who work in the field are forced to keep up not only with ever-evolving best practices but with a very dynamic business and regulatory environment. In both clinical and administrative management of an inpatient service, the ability to effect swift but deliberate changes and rapid improvement has become a necessity, sometimes determining the survival of a service. How to do this well, and how to lead this well, is not taught in medical schools and is only emerging as an offering in business schools.

We will share our experiences with using lean as a continuous improvement and performance engineering technology to effect rapid changes within a relatively large inpatient psychiatric service of a public general hospital. Table 7.1 lists some major changes in the functioning of our inpatient services we were able to effect. We will describe these efforts in detail in this chapter, hopefully generating further ideas how to use lean for transformational change in inpatient psychiatric settings.

Chapter 1 introduced the basic principles and the history of lean. The "burning platform" or need for change driving the use of lean has also been described elsewhere. We feel, however, that we need to provide the reader with some context introducing the service and outlining the circumstances under which the lean initiatives took place.

The Background Story

A fatality in the psychiatric emergency room of the hospital in 2008 placed the hospital and its psychiatric services in the spotlight and highlighted shortcomings in the resources dedicated and in the provision of psychiatric care within the emergency and inpatient psychiatric services. A new management team was faced with the task to review, reform, and redefine the services in compliance with a court settlement agreement reached with the U.S. Department of Justice, and others. The challenge

Table 7.1 **Summary of Inpatient Service Improvements Using Lean**

Issue	Before	After
Child inpatient service occupancy rate	50%	80%
Patient flow	bottlenecks	Improved patient flow
Staff resource utilization	Staff downtimes	Flexible use of staff resources
Care model	Medical: limited active participation of patients in team meetings	Recovery: regular active participation of patients in team meetings

included retaining old and recruiting new staff and leading them to share a single mission and vision for the department, changing culture, and adopting and establishing best clinical practices, all without reduction in service capacity and while maintaining a safe and stable therapeutic milieu.

The inpatient psychiatric services moved to a new physical plant, and the staff increased in number. The service was organized in nine separate psychiatric units with a total of 205 beds (45 of them for children and adolescents). The new leadership made a conscious decision to adopt lean as a main vehicle for the changes to be implemented, the improvement system already espoused by the hospital's corporate parent organization. Unique to this effort was the scale and depth of use of lean thinking and tools in the behavioral health setting, ranging from identifying and prioritizing problem areas, to engaging staff in creative thinking and collaboration, to coming up with solutions, to implementing innovations and measuring their impact.

The Bird's-Eye View

Some of us writing this story were initiated in lean through participating in a vertical value stream mapping (VVSM) event, which identified and outlined the priorities for action over the course of a year. For any lean activity, a necessary step is defining metrics, which quantify the outcomes expected from the improvement work. Measurable indicators are used to establish baselines ("current state") and monitor if the targeted improvements are achieved. In the inpatient services we posited that the most value for our customer (the patient), is created by quality, safety, and growth in service capacity (without expansion of resources). We decided to measure quality as rates of recidivism (repeat admissions within 15 days of discharge), inpatient length of stay, and patient satisfaction. We defined safety as rates of restraint episodes per 100 patient days and rates of assault incidents per 100 patient days. As indicators for growth in capacity, we chose the percentage of discharges happening during the weekend and time from decision to admit (admission order in CPEP) to arrival on the inpatient unit.

Looking at our current state metrics and having identified our target state in qualitative and quantitative terms, we mapped the movement of a patient throughout the continuum of services the department offered and identified the areas in need of lean action with highest potential for achieving our targets.

For the inpatient psychiatric services, these areas can be grouped in three broad categories:

- Patient flow and related processes
- Clinical processes driving care delivery (assessment, treatment planning, discharge planning)
- Medical and nursing care culture within the inpatient psychiatric service

Rapid improvement events (RIEs), projects, and "just do its" were planned depending on the scope of improvement needed and were sequenced in time.

Staff Insights

This value stream mapping was my first experience with lean. I was asked to participate in the event 2 months into my tenure at the hospital. I had driven a Toyota but knew nothing of lean, and at the time lean concepts were not covered by the hospital or departmental orientation (this has since changed). To me, quality management meant a hospital department and performance improvement was what people from the Joint Commission (a national body promoting health care standards and monitoring health care organizations on their adherence to the standards) liked to talk about. I was passionate about clinical work and doing it right but was not aware that performance, science and engineering could be used in the same sentence. On a Monday I entered a room full of the "who's who" in the department. For the following 3 days everyone collaborated on a first-name basis in both mapping the patient care process flow and in strategic planning. Two senseis managed and channeled the enthusiasm. Every idea found its way to a place on a huge board, leading to what ultimately became the vision of the department. The creative energy and level of engagement in the room were nothing like I had experienced before in any leadership meeting or retreat I had attended. There was a sense of shared ownership and empowerment, a free yet managed flight of ideas steered skillfully into a concise and self-conscious, 1-year, phased target state for the department

The Patient Flow Problem

The VVSM identified transitions in patient care as areas in need of improvement. It highlighted a series of bottlenecks in patient flow throughout the service continuum within the department. The Behavioral Health Services (BHS) department was, theoretically, well positioned to provide an integrated and seamless flow of behavioral health services along its continuum of service settings. It operated a Comprehensive Psychiatric Emergency Program (CPEP), an inpatient psychiatric service, and outpatient clinics. However the services were operating in relative silos with poor communication between them.

There was lack of integration in clinical processes and documentation between CPEP and the inpatient service to allow for rapid stabilization of patients ("customer value"). The time from decision to admit (made in CPEP) to actual arrival of the patient to an inpatient floor ranged anywhere from 1 to 6 hours; the average stay in CPEP for an adult patient was 9.6 hours. Accurate information about bed availability was hard to come by, and as a result, it was hard to know if a patient could be sent upstairs from the CPEP. The bed assignment process was opaque, cumbersome and time consuming.

On the outflow side of the equation, patients were staying on the inpatient services upward of 27 days on average; they would rarely leave in the morning on the day of discharge and discharges would routinely occur after the 4 p.m. shift change. No discharges happened on the weekends. Treatment teams on the inpatient units produced referral packets late (after 12 days of inpatient stay on average) and often the referrals to the outpatient department (OPD) were incomplete or missing essential information. As a result, despite 15 elements identified in the process, hand off of care from inpatient to outpatient setting was poor, with patients not being seen for intake in OPD on the day of discharge from the inpatient unit as expected. Staff in both inpatient and outpatient clinical areas were frustrated with each other. Prolonged inpatient stays and difficulty securing outpatient intake appointments created a systemic "back up," resulting in higher CPEP census, longer stays in CPEP and more frequent calls for Emergency Medical Services diversion to other hospitals. Many clinical processes varied from provider to provider and there was no established standard of work. In summary, the system was set up to "push" patients along the continuum, rather than "pull" them (a lean goal) toward the next level of care.

We tackled these problems with a series of rapid improvement events focusing on patient flow and the barriers to it. Interdisciplinary teams were brought together from contingent clinical areas (psychiatric emergency room and inpatient service; inpatient and outpatient services) and charged with creating solutions and monitoring plans to accelerate flow and improve patient experience. The clinicians directly involved with patient care walked out of these events with a new appreciation and understanding for the efforts of their counterparts in other clinical areas, and out of the intense and exhausting event sessions, new and lasting collaborations emerged.

One example of our improving through the use of lean to address issues in patient flow and related processes has been the transformation in the delivery of the child and adolescent acute psychiatric inpatient services in the hospital. The 2009 VVSM identified the need to reconfigure the structure and delivery of child and adolescent acute behavioral health services (CPEP, extended observation unit, and walk-in clinic). At the time, the existing arrangement was that children and adolescents were seen in CPEP, where a clinical area was designated for that use. A team of child-trained clinicians was available in CPEP but was not fully staffed and shared responsibilities for attending to adult patients. At times of high demand, CPEP would often call for help from child-trained clinicians from other areas, disrupting their workflow and creating tensions between staff. There were no standards or procedures for direct admission of children to the psychiatric units from other emergency rooms or inpatient services, causing delays in making decisions about who to admit and straining relationships with other providers. At the same time,

---

Staff Insights

The thing that I remember the most about being a part of a lean event was the optimism of the conversation. Public mental health is an especially difficult field to work in and sometimes employees become mired in a sort of cynicism that eventually impacts morale. It is easy to lose sight of the importance of the services that we provide when we are too focused on the challenges that we face. Having a perspective on the movements that we will make as an organization helped me understand my role in a more holistic way, which I was able to take back to my coworkers on the inpatient units. I was glad to be asked to participate because I think it demonstrated that leadership values employee input and empowerment. I think that what was important about my being asked to join in the event was that it created a connection between different levels of the system—administration and unit-level employees—so that we are all truly working together to achieve the same end. I have worked for much smaller organizations where the solutions naturally incorporated all levels of the system—simply because the small size of the group. In all the public mental health settings in which I have been employed, and this is especially true in New York, the systems have been much more bureaucratic and inefficient. Solutions to problems are slow in coming and the agencies are not able to adapt to the quickly changing times. It is refreshing to see a more efficient and constantly evolving system that fully utilizes the talents of all the employees function in such a large hospital.

the child and adolescent psychiatric inpatient service utilized about only 50% of its census capacity and walk-ins were seen in a newly established Central Intake Unit (CIU). The CIU was situated in close proximity to the CPEP but was staffed by clinicians from the outpatient clinic, who would travel several floors down to get to the CIU. Clinicians covering walk-ins would stand by during down times in CIU and would not be available to the outpatient clinic, creating inefficient use of staff time. The patients, who were used to having their walk-in visits in the outpatient clinic, had a hard time finding and utilizing the CIU, resulting in even more downtime for the CIU. The redirection of patients showing up for walk-in visits in the outpatient clinic caused them inconvenience and care delays. There was dissatisfaction on the part of patients and referring agencies with the accessibility of services and a growing sense of futility on the part of clinicians working in the outpatient clinics.

The value stream map provided for a 6-month project to analyze existing service provision capacity and design, research service needs in the catchment area and the borough, and come up with a strategy for service development for the child and adolescent acute services. The value stream map, a series of activities leading to "gates," or review points, laid out the order of all activities needed to reach the target state. The map was a huge creature, a large grid covering a wall with post-its. Across the top of the map we identified supplies and customers of child and adolescent services, as well as the "core team" of individuals who would have responsibility for completing any of the project tasks. At the far, bottom left side of the map, we established the date by which we wanted the whole project to be finished. Along the bottom row of the map we put a description of the purpose of and process for periodic reviews that we would conduct and a description of a "freeze point," a point in the flow of activities that we would place on the map in which we would "lock" decisions and status. The freeze points would help us not second guess our work; a freeze point placed on the map meant we would agree to go forward and not re-do work to date. This was a new concept for us—how many times have we worked projects over and over and never reached the goal? Our sensei taught us not to "let perfect be the enemy of good."

To fill in the map, we identified all of the steps, in sequence that must be completed to reach our target state for child and adolescent services. Actions, or tasks, were placed in descending order on post-its below the primary person on the core team who was accountable for completing the task. To support the task's primary person, we identified all of the other members of the core team who would have a role in the task. For each task we noted, on the right side of the map, any standard work that would be produced as a result of the task as well as any RIEs that would be required. We selected about 5 points—the "gates"—at which we would do comprehensive status reviews during the course of the project. For each gate, we set dates for these reviews and specific deliverables that had to be completed before the implementation team could enter each gate. The deliverables were those things we would need to bring to each review to evaluate our work. We also established the outputs expected from each review—evidence of completed tasks, documented standard work, research findings with conclusions. The VVSM team then agreed on which gates were "freeze points," locking our work, and which outputs were essential before we could move through the gate. This "go/no-go" approach to each gate recognized that if certain conditions weren't met, the subsequent activities would be suboptimized and result in the waste of unnecessary rework. The discipline to adhere what we established as inputs to, and outputs of each gate would be challenging. A sense of, "let's just get this done..." or "at least it is so much better than it used to be..." is hard to resist when a new process for project management was being asked of us and was, well, new and not yet proven. We filled in dates for all of the tasks between each major review, and the map was complete and real work could begin.

A workgroup, including clinical leaders across disciplines and clinical areas within child and adolescent services, was created to conduct the research and perform the analysis. As the workgroup took on its task, it found it efficient to divide into several subgroups. One subgroup took on researching the options for the most efficient provision of emergency services. A second workgroup looked at partial hospital and intensive outpatient programs and the feasibility of offering these services as part of the acute service continuum. A third subgroup looked at the direct admissions process and the walk-in visit process.

All subgroups met weekly and worked independently. They assembled the results of their research and analysis in a pre-agreed-upon presentation format. The final product was reviewed and edited by the whole workgroup and represented a strategic vision of the makeup of child and adolescent acute behavioral health services to be offered by the department. The workgroup team members presented this shared vision to department leadership and representatives of the regional New York State Office of Mental Health. The project was organized and ran based on lean tools. It

---

Staff Insights

It was exhausting and exhilarating at the same time, as well as emotionally draining because we were taking on several challenges at once that at times seemed to be unsolvable. The team was a good one and the focus was, as it should have been, on what would work in a practical sense in the real world of our units. I was glad to be involved in planning for the outpatient clinics so that I could present our strengths and weaknesses and be part of a change process that would make sense for us. It was also gratifying to be involved in the effort to tackle service delivery challenges across the different child programs. Sharing perspectives and ideas was invaluable. It allowed us to retain a sense of control over our work and to work together as a cohesive team.

Staff Insights

I remember being energized by the project (exploring CPEP options), by the fact that I was included in it and by the research I did for the project. I was pleased to be invited as a participant and it felt validating to be included in discussions about the future directions our service was taking.

---

had several important intangible benefits. It inspired and energized clinical staff and leadership to creatively collaborate in informing decisions about the strategic development of the service. It promoted the idea that change is needed and gave staff a sense of control and direction in bringing it about.

Now that we had envisioned what direction we wanted to take, we were ready to start change implementation. We were ready for a rapid improvement event (RIE). An RIE is meant to generate and test solutions to an identified inefficient process (eliminate waste). We put much thought into selecting the team for this event. It included a representative of child and adolescent behavioral health leadership from the corporate central office, the chief of the hospital's pediatric service (as "fresh eyes"), child clinicians across disciplines including psychiatry, social work and psychology from CPEP, the inpatient and outpatient services. The eight-member team had as its reason for action "a perception of barriers to access to child and adolescent behavioral health care services both within the department and from the community." The identified initial state included complaints to regulatory agencies about access to our services, length of stay in CPEP for children increasing and a walk-in clinic with increased utilization of services without an optimal structure or resources to support it. The target state envisioned seamless referrals to child and adolescent acute services, child-friendly CPEP processes, a shorter length of stay for children in CPEP, and smarter and more flexible resource allocation in all child services.

THE CHILD AND ADOLESCENT SUPPORT TEAM

The team came up with the idea of a cross-disciplinary Child and Adolescent Support Team (CAST) to be assembled of licensed clinicians, who would dedicate 2 hours of their time per week to be available at a short notice. Clinicians were asked to plan their week so that these predetermined 2 hours in their weekly schedule were not dedicated to patient care, but to administrative or documentation tasks so that if they were pulled on, patient care would not be disrupted. The team would be deployed at the request of service areas overwhelmed by the inflow of patients to aid with assessments and disposition planning. A scheduling template for the CAST was tested in rapid experiments and determined to support the CAST scope and time of operations. The RIE team met with the supervisors of service areas to determine the most likely situations when the CAST might be called on for help.

As part of the rapid experiments the RIE team also assessed staff's willingness to participate as a CAST member and determined that if the innovation was to succeed, then expectations for time commitment and predictability would be important. The RIE team created a standard of work for the CAST based on the rapid experiment outcomes. In their shared insights, the RIE team members found the exchange of ideas and discussions illuminating "the big picture," as well as hearing historical background of specific clinical areas helpful. They were pleased with their understanding and discussion of clinical units, with the gemba walk (visiting and observing the clinical areas work flow), the open discussions, and having "fresh eyes" on the team. They felt hindered by "talking on too much," (versus "doing"), by what they saw as an insufficient ability to think out of the box, and by what they saw as too much focus on one clinical area (namely, CPEP).

Following the RIE, we completed the reorganization of the acute services with several "just do its." We created a standard of work for direct admissions to the inpatient service. We designated a phone line to be the "referral hotline" operated by a direct referral coordinator, retraining a clerical staff with this new job function and redistributing other functions among existing clerical staff. We mounted an outreach effort through the department of social work to facilities and agencies that by the nature of the services they offered seemed our most likely collaborators and customers. We continued to track and report our "confirmed state" data and were able to close out the RIE after 6 months of consistently meeting our targets. The CAST was able to successfully reduce bottlenecks in staff resources and address peaks in service demand in clinical areas of the child and adolescent BHS in a most flexible way, allowing as a byproduct cross-training of clinical staff and breaking up some of the existing silos between disciplines and clinical areas. The utilization rate of our inpatient child and adolescent service census capacity (previously at 50%) rose to an average of 80% and continues to trend upward toward an optimal goal of 85%.

The Clinical Process Redesign

As we noted in the introduction to this chapter, the second broad category of processes on the inpatient services identified for intervention were the clinical processes driving care delivery (assessment, treatment planning, and discharge planning).

Our main reason for action here was the gap we identified between our existing clinical processes and procedures and the core clinical philosophy of patient-centered and wellness- and recovery-oriented care we had adopted. As directed by the value stream map, we sequenced our lean activities to match the flow of our clinical processes The assessment process was first in this sequence to be reviewed in a series of RIEs. We recognized that we lacked a standard of work for the assessment process,

---

Lessons Learned

Lean is about eliminating waste wherever it is found by utilizing the people that understand the process. Planning for change is accomplished with respect for the individual staff, who are involved in critical analysis of the day-to-day work process, catalyzing them to become the agents of change. This is the formula for sustained improvement.

---

that there was fragmented communication between clinical team members, and that the assessments were not getting completed in a timely manner. We mapped the assessment workflow and revealed 12 discrete steps with many professional disciplines working in silos.

The first RIE on inpatient assessment was able to reduce the 12 major steps in the assessment workflow to 4.

Three major obstacles to the target state were identified through analyzing the gap between our current state and the target state. These obstacles were limitations of the existing electronic medical record, the lack of true team work, and ineffective staff orientation and training. To get to the root cause for each of these obstacles and generate solutions, teams used a lean tool called the "five whys." (see Table 7.2).

The five whys can help in drilling down to the root causes of enduring problems impacting the quality and quantity of the work process. Similar to the Socratic questioning used in cognitive behavioral therapy, the team runs the problem statement through a series of why questions. The answer at each level is subjected to the same process. The idea is that by the fifth pass one has moved beyond symptoms to a "root cause" and this is the true "gap" for which a solution needs to be identified. The solution is stated in an "If we," "then we" format, ensuring that the solution suggested matches the problem identified—as opposed to some other interesting but unrelated problem (see Table 7.3). It is a balanced process designed to prevent one from diverging on to the enticing but impractical path of having an "academic" discussion about the problem and losing sight of the task at hand—namely, generating a solution.

Using the "five whys," lack of teamwork was identified to be the result of disciplinary silos and turf wars and a culture based on fear of losing one's job that came, at least in part, from the emotional toll of sustained oversight by multiple agencies due to our burning platform. Expectations of accountability were experienced as punitive. Failures in training and orientation were found to be rooted in assumptions that new staff could "hit the ground running," resulting in a perception of disconnect between management and staff. The root causes identified during the brainstorming process of the "five whys" were staffs' attempt to articulate the complexity of the problems they were facing, colored by the emotions they experienced

Table 7.2 **The "Five Whys" Tool Used in the Assessments Rapid Improvement Event**

What	Why	Why	Why	Why	Why
Qmed not user friendly	Fragmented process built into design	Line staff not included in design of Qmed	Culture of top-down management	Leadership was under pressure as a result of incidents, lawsuits, and regulatory agencies	Result of past poor practice in planning, in staffing, and in using tools
No true team approach	Disciplines working in silos	Discipline turf wars	Culture based on fear of losing job	Administration and staff feel punished	Because of attempts at accountability that were experienced as scapegoating
Orientation and ongoing training to BHS ineffective	Needs assessment for staff not completed	Assumption that licensed staff can hit ground running and work as a team	Unrealistic expectations about difficulty of adopting to environment here at HHC	Administration disconnected from staff and clinical environment	Administration focused on regulatory needs rather than staff and patient needs

in processing the urgency and pace of changes. It was evident that staff felt overwhelmed, taxed, and at times resentful.

Recognizing the reality of poor staff morale, a 9-month engagement project was undertaken by a group of talented and dedicated staff members, who went about polling staff in the department—directly and indirectly via "idea trees" (boards where yellow stickers like leaves on a tree could be left anonymously throughout the hospital—see Figure 7.1)—on their ideas of what needs to change to improve engagement and morale. The results of the project were rolled out in a department-wide "town hall meeting" with management's commitment to implement the best suggestions.

Enhancements to the electronic medical record, development of a "just culture" that promotes accountability and teamwork free of fear and retaliation by managers, with regular discussions of staff training needs, were the solution approaches generated out of this discovery process. A practice of regular Town Hall meetings with

Table 7.3 **The "If We, Then We" Format Used in the Assessments Rapid Improvement Event**

Gap	If We	Then We
Qmed not user friendly	Involve staff in designing user-friendly tools and training…	Have needs-based training and tools that enhance patient care.
No true team approach	Practiced "just culture"…	Have accountability and enhanced teamwork free from fear.
Orientation ongoing training to BHS ineffective	Encourage leadership and line staff to work together to take ownership of outcomes through a regular discussion of needs…	Decrease both staff confusion and future incidents through open discussion and ongoing training.

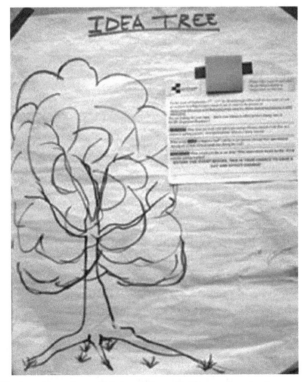

Figure 7.1 Idea tree is used to solicit input from staff on a given topic.

all staff and departmental leadership was instituted. Electronic anonymous opinion polling (clickers) and real-time feedback visuals were used to present and process anonymous staff feedback on various topics. The monthly department newsletter also communicated relevant and timely information.

The solutions approaches generated to address the root causes to assessment problems that were identified by using the "five whys" included development of key questions for a structured interview that reduced redundancy between discipline assessments, design of a visual erase board that would enhance the understanding of the standard of work, and pursuing enhancements to the EMR. Standard work is a key product of rapid experiments and the success of lean sustainment. It defines the boundaries of a task, names who performs it and most importantly how it is to be done. Standard work enables consistency of performance for repeated tasks and reduces variability that leads to waste and poor task or product outcomes. It specifies the pace at which a service or function must be produced to meet demand, or "takt time." The standard work created by the team reflected findings the team made through time observations, in which the team was able to confirm how long each step in the process took and which resources were used for each process. With this information, the team was able to use real data to eliminate unnecessary tasks, level the workload across staff, and create a staffing plan designed to enable the new, more efficient assessment process based on the cadence of patient needs. A completion plan was set for the various individuals who would spearhead the resulting recommendations and target quality metrics were set for the completion of all disciplines' assessments.

Within 5 months of the RIE select units had reached the goal of timely assessments. Assessment of psychiatric risks was embedded in the assessment process and started driving treatment planning. Table 7.4 highlights our outcomes following the RIE.

The work on improving the assessment process did not stop at this. We had several other passes with RIEs, focusing on reassessments and how they inform formulation and treatment plan updates. The RIE team in one of the RIEs created a diagram to illustrate their vision the reassessment process (Figure 7.2).

A restructured medical record entry—the "weekly note" came into being as the result of one of the RIE generated solution approaches. The new standard of work for psychiatrists defined this note as the place to summarize a patient's progress in treatment and to review significant events in the course of care for the past week. Clinical observations and history gathered over the course of the week would register to inform changes in formulation and diagnosis. Since its introduction, this note has been much appreciated by clinicians from all disciplines in need of an up-to-date brief clinical summary. The note was particularly helpful to weekend/holiday-covering house physician staff.

Another area where lean proved very helpful was the creation and integration of a behavior support team (BST) in the inpatient service assessment and treatment

Table 7.4 **Assessments RIE outcomes tracking table**

Indicator	Metric	Baseline (9 units total)	Target (7w & 4W)	60-Day (7w & 4W)	90-Day (7w & 4W)	120-Day (7w & 4W)	150 Day (7w & 4W)
Safety	Initial INPT High-riskassessment within 8 hours	Adult Suicide = 98% Adult Violence = 98% Adult Sexual = 94% Child Suicide = 98% Child Violence = 13% Child Sexual = 87%	Adult = 95% Child = 95%	Adult Suicide = 100% Adult Violence = 100% Adult Sexual = 97% Child Suicide = 80% Child Violence = 80% Child Sexual = 100%	Adult Suicide = 97% Adult Violence = 100% Adult Sexual = 100% Child Suicide = 100% Child Violence = 100% Child Sexual = 100%	Adult Suicide = 100% Adult Violence = 91% Adult Sexual = 100% Child Suicide = 75% Child Violence = 83% Child Sexual = 92%	Adult Suicide = 100% Adult Violence = 100% Adult Sexual = 97% Child Suicide = 100% Child Violence = 100% Child Sexual = 100%
Quality	Nursing assessment within 8 hours	Adult = 76% Child = 89%	Adult = 85% Child = 95%	Adult = 83% Child = 100%	Adult = 100% Child = 100%	Adult = 100% Child = 93%	Adult = 97% Child = 100%
Quality	Psychiatrist assessment within 24 hours	Adult = 58% Child = 70%	Adult = 85% Child = 85%	Adult = 66% Child = 100%	Adult = 80% Child = 88%	Adult = 84% Child = 87%	Adult = 86% Child = 83%
Quality	Psychosocial assessment within 72 hours	Adult = 76 Child = 20	Adult = 85% Child = 85%	Adult = 83% Child = 20	Adult = 94% Child = 100%	Adult = 92% Child = 93%	Adult = 81% Child = 100%
Quality	Medical assessment within 72 hours	Adult = retrieve Child = retrieve	Adult = 95% Child = 90%	Adult = 86% Child = retrieve	Adult = 94.5% Child = 87.5%	Adult = 96% Child = 100%	Adult = 94% Child = 75%
Safety	Total incidents Q1	340 (113 per month = 12.5 per unit)	<30610% reduction (106 per month = 11 per unit)	Adult = 6 Child = 7	Adult = 7 Child = 5	Adult = 3 Child = 14	Adult = 8 Child = 14
Safety	Reportable incidents Q1	113 per month = 40 per unit	<920% reduction (3 per month = 33 per unit)	zero for both	Adult = Zero Child = 1	Adult = Zero Child = Zero	Adult = Zero Child = 1

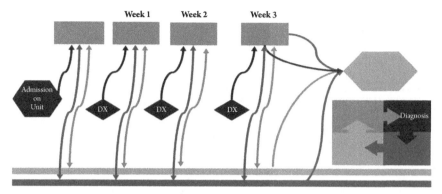

Figure 7.2 Diagram representing the reassessment flow within the treatment continuum as conceptualized by the RIE team.

workflow. The BST was conceived as a way to address the need of advanced behavior assessment, management, and treatment planning for patients with particularly challenging behaviors. It included behaviorally trained psychologists, a nurse, an occupational therapist, and behavior analysts, who would observe and analyze behavior of referred patients and aid the treatment team in developing individualized behavior plans or positive behavior support plans, targeting the problem behaviors. These plans would then guide interactions between staff and the patient. Lean thinking and project management allowed us within a short period of time to create a working structure and process where there were none before and include the BST in the intervention armamentarium of treatment teams. A simplified diagram of the referral and work flow for the BST is presented in Figure 7.3. The BST collaboration led to marked reductions in violence and the need for restrictive interventions.

Nursing tools for the assessment of risk for suicide, violence, and self-harm were also developed as part of the solution approaches to improving risk assessments, recommended in the RIE. Here we made use of a lean project (as previously noted, projects are used for addressing problems of larger scope, requiring more resources and/or time than a single RIE). We created a work group with the service director as a process owner, a team leader, and a balance of members who participated in the assessment RIEs and some who brought fresh eyes and experience to the task at hand. Within months this group searched the literature, developed or revised policies, and chose or created support tools to guide decisions around clinical assessment and response to psychiatric risk. Collaborative relationships, mutual respect, and cohesion were some of the lasting byproducts of the group's work. One participant in the assessment RIEs fondly remembers being upset at being recruited for the event, as she could not understand what could be so important as to pull her away from her clinical responsibilities for 5 days. After her initial misgivings,

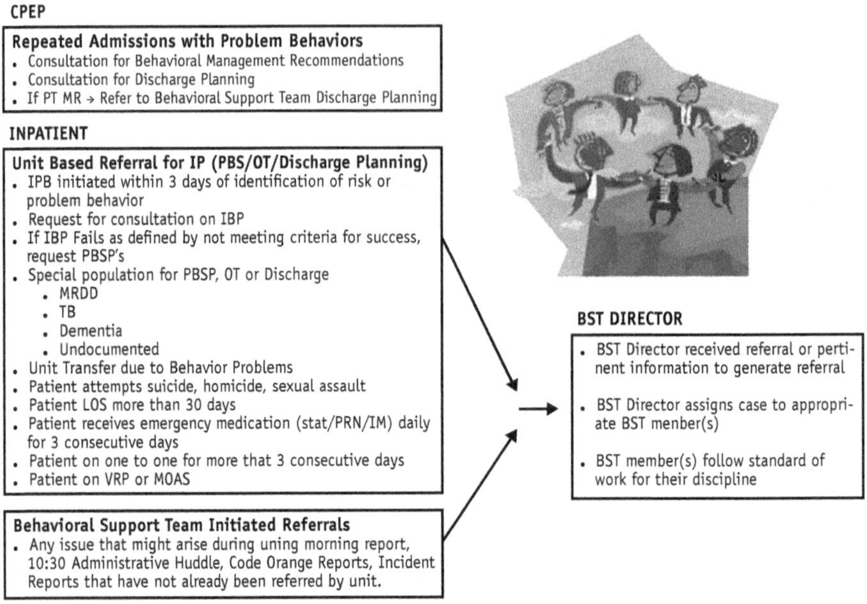

CPEP

Repeated Admissions with Problem Behaviors
- Consultation for Behavioral Management Recommendations
- Consultation for Discharge Planning
- If PT MR → Refer to Behavioral Support Team Discharge Planning

INPATIENT

Unit Based Referral for IP (PBS/OT/Discharge Planning)
- IPB initiated within 3 days of identification of risk or problem behavior
- Request for consultation on IBP
- If IBP Fails as defined by not meeting criteria for success, request PBSP's
- Special population for PBSP, OT or Discharge
  - MRDD
  - TB
  - Dementia
  - Undocumented
- Unit Transfer due to Behavior Problems
- Patient attempts suicide, homicide, sexual assault
- Patient LOS more than 30 days
- Patient receives emergency medication (stat/PRN/IM) daily for 3 consecutive days
- Patient on one to one for more that 3 consecutive days
- Patient on VRP or MOAS

Behavioral Support Team Initiated Referrals
- Any issue that might arise during uning morning report, 10:30 Administrative Huddle, Code Orange Reports, Incident Reports that have not already been referred by unit.

BST DIRECTOR
- BST Director received referral or pertinent information to generate referral
- BST Director assigns case to appropriate BST menber(s)
- BST member(s) follow standard of work for their discipline

Figure 7.3 Diagram of the Behavioral Support Team (BST) referral process and work flow.

she found she did like the process and the idea of trying to make things better and appreciated her involvement as line staff. She felt proud of the products the team developed and stayed committed to the idea of continuous improvement.

The process owner for the assessment work group felt very proud of the products they created, including assessment policies, procedures, and screening tools. She felt the work had set the foundation for the inpatient service to foster a patient-centered treatment culture, naturally evolving from the more coercive treatment practices of the past. She also felt that the productive outcome of the project had enhanced her overall professional confidence.

The next focus for lean transformation, as identified in our value stream map, was the treatment process itself. We sequenced several RIEs to address key elements: diagnostic decision support and treatment algorithms, treatment practices, and discharge planning. Diagnostic and treatment algorithms for depression, schizophrenia, and bipolar disorder, our the three most common admission diagnoses, were created and tested in rapid experiments to obtain staff feedback. A repeat admissions review committee was created to provide in-depth analysis of readmissions of patients who rapidly return to the hospital. The committee was to assist teams in developing alternative discharge plans for patients with repeat admissions. It was comprised of representatives of all disciplines in supervisory roles on the service, who would meet with treatment teams to review the circumstances of a readmission.

Using the process we followed for assessment transformation we next tackled treatment planning and discharge planning. An RIE planned and kicked off changes in targeted units, followed by a work group overseeing the detailing and implementation of changes over the course of 6 months (a lean project) on all units. Work groups on treatment planning and on discharge planning were assembled from representatives of all relevant disciplines (social work, psychology, nursing, psychiatry, internal medicine, therapeutic rehabilitation, and peer counselors). Group members were line staff with firsthand experience and intimate knowledge of the clinical processes under review. Each work group had a team leader and a process owner. The team leader was a clinical supervisor (middle manager) of a discipline thought to be a main stakeholder in the clinical process (e.g., psychology for treatment planning and social work for discharge planning). The process owner was a senior clinical leader in the department (e.g., assistant chief of service for treatment planning and director of social work for discharge planning). The main deliverables for the workgroups were any policy changes needed to codify new practices; discipline-specific, detailed standards of work to describe and guide workflow; any changes to the medical record (electronic or paper) needed to accommodate new processes and practices; training content and materials for staff with measure of competency achieved; and metrics and methods to measure compliance with new practices and processes. The workgroups met independently, usually weekly. A process owners' meeting was held periodically to inform each other of the workgroups progress, exchange information, and coordinate issues cutting across workgroups. The workgroup product was submitted for review and approval by the Top Management Team (TMT), comprised of department discipline heads and executive leadership. Approved product were forwarded for training and implementation and metrics was forwarded to the quality management department for data collection, monitoring, and reporting.

Staff Insights

What worked very well was the interdisciplinary composition of the team, mirroring the composition of a treatment team. We faced the same challenges a treatment team faces, with members with different levels of enthusiasm and engagement and a different pace of work. Working together, we were able to overcome these differences and began to like each other as we got to know each other. The most exciting part of the work was creating an enactment of a treatment planning meeting to be used as a teaching tool. Having a peer counselor on the team to bring in the patient perspective, and to refocus us when needed, was invaluable. They also did a superb job as our pretend patient during the enactment. We all felt very proud of the products we created, and I am sure each of us brought new ideas and enthusiasm back to our own treatment teams.

Lessons Learned

No single lean tool, event, or intervention "fixes" a problem or process. "Continuous" is a key word in understanding how lean works and what it takes.

We saw the lean project tool as the method of choice to effect changes in multiple clinical processes over a relatively short period of time. The workgroup idea allowed for a parallel process of change in several areas at the same time. It had its inherent challenges in that we had to ask a number of clinicians to dedicate extra time and effort beyond their regular clinical duties and their colleagues to provide coverage for the time spent in meetings. We had to draw from the same pool of forward-thinking, change interested and engaged staff to balance the composition of the workgroup teams in setting them up for success. The intensity and fast pace of the work proved taxing to some and invigorating to others.

TRAINING AND COACHING

We have had several passes at improving the same clinical processes to achieve additional incremental changes. Every new event finds new waste to eliminate and a new level of improvement to layer on foundations built by previous lean efforts. The lean transformation of our treatment planning process is a good example. We took the treatment planning workgroup products, as approved by the BH Senior Management Team, and mounted a massive training effort to disseminate the new practice expectations to all clinical staff on the inpatient service. We did this by conducting training sessions on all shifts and distributing DVD recordings and printed materials. We followed with having members of the treatment planning workgroup observe and rate treatment team meetings, identify underperforming teams and to offer them support. After an initial burst of improvement and enthusiasm, over time, with staff changes and competing priorities, treatment planning practices seemed to regress to the mean of the past, over the course of 6 months. Our own monitoring, as well as that being conducted by DOJ, noted wide variability in treatment team practices and performance.

It requires ongoing efforts in the areas of processes and people to sustain system changes. Some of the common pitfalls of improvement initiatives, which we think were at play in our treatment planning project, have been described by Thomas Choi.[1] We experienced alienation of line leaders—involvement and improvement being seen as interfering with their performance objective. We also had clinicians seeing improvement as a management program—bypassing workers. Finally, we may have had the workgroup improvement team identified as "special forces," thereby building resentment in treatment team clinicians. The insufficient resource allocation to the initial effort may have created the perception of "there we go again"—another intermittent stop-go initiative with questionable commitment from leadership.

We registered these observations in a new "reason for action" and "initial state" and developed a new lean project, this time targeting standardization of treatment planning practices and adherence to the best practice model, established by the treatment planning workgroup in their training video. We assembled a group of treatment planning "coaches." These were clinicians from all disciplines, recommended by discipline leaders based on performance in practice, for their use of wellness and recovery philosophy of care and demonstrated knowledge and skills in treatment planning. The staff selected as coaches passed a "coach aptitude test" querying them on principles of recovery, their knowledge of our identified best practice, and their understanding of what constitutes a well-functioning treatment team. The group of 23 coaches (one for each treatment team and two substitutes) started meeting once per week. First it established a standard of work for coaches and team leaders vis-à-vis the lean project. Then the group researched, adapted, and adopted a set of team performance measures to monitor treatment team process and function (including a patient satisfaction component). It developed ratings to be used by treatment teams to measure coach's impact and teams' satisfaction with coaching. As the coaching process began, the group continued to meet regularly to share observations and establish ongoing conventions for feedback practice and language, with a focus on consistency and clarity in expectations. The coaches' effort was circumscribed to 2 to 3 hours per week, and discipline leaders made a commitment upfront to provide for the coaches' clinical coverage. The duration of the lean project was estimated to last 12 to 16 months, and at the time of this writing it is still ongoing. We established as a target of 90% performance rating on the team performance measures we devised and estimated that given the initial state variability in team performance, we would need a dedicated coaching resource for at least a year to achieve our targets. We would then re-evaluate the coaching and monitoring resources needed to sustain improvement. We tied the team performance measures to departmental service quality indicators and began tracking and trending them with feedback to treatment teams and coaches.

We have already identified positive energy emerging and spreading from the coaching project. The staff engaged in coaching enjoyed the validation of their skills and the opportunity to share them with others. They can see their observations and opinions driving change and making a difference. They benefit from the sharing and learning with like-minded and caring professionals. They seed the department with a network of engaged and personally connected professionals, with a sense of community, ready and driving for change. Each of the coaching clinicians at the same time returns to a treatment team of their own and inevitably influences their teammates' attitudes and practices.

We approached staff that had participated in the treatment planning projects to share their experiences. A team member invited to participate in the RIE only weeks after employment in the hospital felt it had been a difficult experience. While recognizing the benefits of the exposure, understanding the particular emphasis on treatment planning in this hospital took some time. She felt more effective in the workgroup project, which followed the RIE, as she now had a better understanding of the overall history of the department. There was a clear sense of pride in the product—the actual process and work flow for treatment planning meetings—and a belief that this was a great foundation on which functioning interdisciplinary teamwork could build upon. She also sensed a great opportunity to work with some very talented members of the work group from other disciplines, with whom she would otherwise not have had any contact.

A member of the discharge planning workgroup was also very pleased with the aftercare planning procedures and documentation developed, replacing the long, confusing, and irrelevant discharge instructions form previously given to patients. The team member was proud of this product, had a sense of ownership, and felt it contributed to improving patient care. Work is continuing with the goal of discharge planning becoming a truly interdisciplinary team effort, and not just a social work task. The workgroup member reflected in retrospect that assessment and treatment planning workgroups were creating parallel products at the same time and may have benefited from combining their efforts—clear opportunity for lean action, identified by a lean novice.

Medical and Nursing Care

Creating and sustaining the changed culture emerging in BHS was by far the most difficult and challenging process. Still, an appropriate environment is essential to ensure that the basic safety requirements for both patient and staff are adequately addressed and intrinsic to the systems in place. A therapeutic milieu needs to include safe staffing ratios, access to basic necessities for patients such as toiletries and linen, and a safe environment for the patient to recover. Keeping order is not treatment. A culture in which there were unmet needs, insufficient patient involvement in treatment planning, less than optimal therapeutic rehabilitation, and a bleak physical environment led to dissatisfaction for staff and patients alike. Perceptions of incompetence and arrogance did little to enhance provision of care.

STAFFING PATTERNS

To begin to address this, nursing staff numbers were gradually increased by 60% to create safe staffing ratios and to deploy an adequate number of appropriately trained and licensed staff as required by the new processes. The VVSM had identified safety as a central theme. As noted earlier in this chapter, through the Gap Analysis the team identified that the critical clinical areas to improve were assessment, medical nursing, medication management, discharge planning, treatment planning, behavioral management, and the environment of care. In other words, all aspects of treatment that are typically provided to a patient admitted to a psychiatric unit from admission to discharge needed review and revision. To achieve this massive overhaul and become a Center of Excellence, with a 5-year goal of providing state of the art care in the safest environment, the team worked on its relationship with DOJ to develop it from a potentially adversarial one to a partnership focused on achieving the targeted state. The team identified four indicators that would help staff measure improvements that ultimately improved the culture of safety: number of significant incidents, use of restraints and STAT psychotropic IM medications, and recidivism. The VVSM process broke down this daunting task into achievable goals over a 1-year period. To achieve the target state, RIEs were conducted in each of the major areas. Some of these RIEs, just do its, and projects have been described elsewhere in this and other chapters but several are worth exploring in depth as they relate very closely to the culture change needed to improve care.

In May 2010 the first Observation RIE took place. The reason for action identified was that despite the multiple levels of nursing observations that are provided to patients, there still have been failures in protecting patients from harm. Through root cause analyses, it was determined that there were several contributing causal factors such as resource allocation, inappropriate use of risk assessments, and failure to follow policy and procedure. The initial state the team identified was that policies and procedures were developed in response to events, the risk screening tools were used as stand-alone justifications for high levels of observation rather than careful clinical evaluation and re-evaluation and that nursing observations were recorded on paper rather than in the electronic medical record utilized for other types of documentation. The gold standard or target state the team strove to achieve would be the development of policy and procedure based on sound clinical standards and careful risk assessment conducted to ensure that proper nursing observation was individualized for each patient, with observations recorded accurately and all staff trained in standard work and policy and procedure.

The team analyzed the waste in the current state of providing care and identified themes that created the gap between the current and targeted states. One example of this waste was easy to identify. Review of the current state of nursing observation forms revealed that there were five different forms all measuring observation. Three other main gaps in reaching the target were that there were multiple levels of observation ordered for one patient causing staff to struggle with understanding the purpose of all the observations and therefore ineffectively monitoring patients. The second gap was that there were too many patients on one-to-one observation level. This created staffing crises in which a few patients utilized a majority of the nursing care hours of the staff assigned to the unit and some patients received less nursing care than their conditions warranted. Finally, the risk assessment tools utilized were too general and lacked sensitivity for symptoms.

Using A3 thinking the team developed a solution for each gap identified. For the RIE focused on observations, methods to reduce duplication of types of observation were listed, risk assessment tools were identified to use as an adjunct to clinical judgment, one-to-one reassessment was structured and time limited, and communication between nurses and physicians was to be vastly improved. After the team identified these solutions they set out to conduct rapid experiments to determine if the solutions suggested would work in reality. The most successful rapid experiment was the consolidation of the five nursing observation forms into one universal form for use with multiple types of observation. The ability to collaborate and develop solutions together helped to ensure that staff would support the recommended changes and had commitment to the new process ensuring sustainment over time.

THE CASE FOR TRAINING

Training, training, training has been one of the solutions identified in every RIE and project. It is important to understand that regardless of type of health-care institution, there is a bell curve that exists regarding clinical expertise of staff assigned to any given unit within the facility. When Kings County increased its staff by more than 60% this bell curve was no longer supportive of the learning environment needed. Those staffs that were providing care to patients that were deemed not meeting expectations separated in various ways from the hospital. Clinicians that remained, along with the new staff hired, were in great need of basic psychiatric training and skills. The nursing department was especially challenged because of a lack of ability to hire seasoned psychiatric nurses probably because of the negative publicity surrounding the hospital and, of course, the usual difficulty in recruiting nurses in New York City. Almost exclusively, new graduates were selected for positions. In December 2010, the first RIE devoted to training was conducted. The burning platform identified in this particular area was that BHS did not have an integrated training department, negatively impacting its ability to effectively communicate current clinical and nonclinical practices and to introduce new standards efficiently and effectively. A silo approach to training was the current state identified. A truly integrated interdisciplinary department equipped to orient and determine competency and needs of staff was the target to reach. Using one of the lean methods to flush out waste a fishbone was developed (presented as Figure 7.4) which identified three critical gaps.

The underlying root cause of each of the gaps was communication deficits. The training team had only a vague understanding of their roles and responsibilities, there was a lack of coordination between department heads and there was no database of information shared between departments inside and outside of BH. By developing a completion plan of just do its, RIEs, and projects the team mapped out the desired training program for new employees. Metrics were developed to ensure

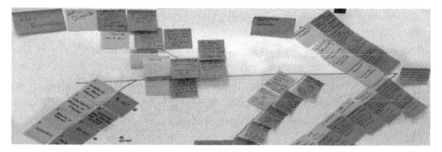

Figure 7.4 Fishbone tool as used in the Training RIE to identify root cause during the gap analysis.

orientation to roles, responsibilities and to measure competency. A database system was designed to manage and track our progress.

The lack of integrated training was very evident in the nursing department of BH. The newly graduated nurses had only school-based experience in both medical and psychiatric care. This lack of specialty training and experience in the medical/surgical area resulted in a struggle to identify and properly assess any comorbidities our patients may have had. A team of physicians and nurses came together to identify and remove the boundaries that hindered good nursing care. The burning platform they identified for this RIE was the fact that medical care was secondary to psychiatric care until a medical emergency occurs. There was also a failure to fully follow or utilize existing policies and procedures for medical and nursing care. As was identified in other RIEs, the medical care provided was crisis driven. Behavioral Health in general was a reactive department, and it was very difficult to care for patients optimally in this type of environment.

Before settling on a target state for this RIE, the RIE team drew their "ideal state," a proactive department with adequate resources where policies and procedures guide holistic care in a standardized format and where that care is delivered in an interdisciplinary manner with streamlined and effective communication. This target state action plan was derived from the waste opportunities identified by the acronym DOWNTIME.

D defects
O overproduction
W waiting
N not best use of talent
T transportation
I inventory
M motion
E extra processing

When the team used these lean concepts, two critical gaps became evident and 36 areas of concern were identified! Those two critical gaps were truly critical for safe patient care. Acute medical situations were often the first time medical concerns were fully addressed, and nursing staff did not optimally carry out lab tests ordered by physicians. Solutions identified by the team were adding desktop nursing queue monitors, which would allow nursing staff to check pending orders and providing user-friendly tools to assist staff in performing targeted assessments of medical issues.

The team developed recipe cards for the three main comorbidities facing psychiatric patients: hypertension, obesity, and diabetes. Armed with these cards, they conducted rapid experiments to determine their usefulness in assisting the nurses in structuring the medical assessment and synthesizing system checks into an overall treatment plan. They also designed and piloted a huddle format to ensure face-to-face communication between changing tours of nursing leadership, psychiatrists, and medical internists that was then piloted.

The last experiment related to medication reconciliation, a very important Joint Commission national patient safety goal. It was found that the medication reconciliation was done intermittently and not reviewed as timely as possible in the pharmacy. The results of this rapid experiment process demonstrated that often system failures are revealed and that the lean process of stripping away waste and redundancy is important to reveal true system failures that would not otherwise easily be identified.

The final completion plan that was developed was determined by the successfully conducted rapid experiments together with the corrections that would be needed to fix the system failures identified. The team also determined the specific metrics that would measure the success of the completion plan. These were a reduction in the fall rate; BMI greater than 30 addressed in the treatment plan; ensuring that patients had follow-up primary care medical appointments if they were diagnosed with hypertension, obesity, or diabetes; and education of all staff in the appropriate activation of the Rapid Response Team (an emergency medical response team for patients experiencing changes in medical status other than cardiopulmonary arrest).

The most important result from an RIE is its impact on the targeted audience or the patient. In this case the difference was apparent in improved patient care, early identification, and treatment of medical conditions by both nursing and medical staff through standardized assessments (recipe cards) improved communication between key players in a patient's treatment(especially between shifts), the development of a phlebotomy team to ensure collection of routine labs, and, finally, pharmacists' timely review of medication reconciliation. These are all significant ways of improving patient safety. One can get a sense of the RIE team's engagement around the issues of patient safety by looking at the RIE work board (Figure 7.5).

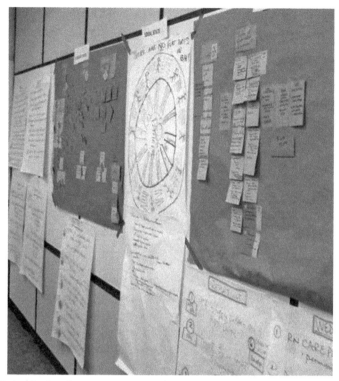

Figure 7.5 Medical and Nursing Care rapid improvement event work board with "ideal state" visual representation (in the center).

CULTURE CHANGE

Culture change is the most difficult change to attain and sustain. It takes years. Our goal (and this is true for any facility paving its way toward excellence in care) must be sustaining the plans identified for each and every improvement made. Countless standards of work are developed, metrics are measured, and goals are perceived to be achieved. Then why is it so striking that the many RIEs, projects, and just do it's over the past few years are eerily similar to those identified at the VSMs for 2011 and 2012? Why are we still focusing on engaging staff to provide a truly integrated model of care in a structured and safe environment that promotes wellness and recovery? Although it seems as if we are at the same milestones identified earlier, we truly are not. The first "true north" hurdles of providing basic safe and therapeutic psychiatric care have been achieved. If we walk our gemba, then our current state supports this. For example, the original RIE for Observation of Patients identified that the process of observation was lacking. The improvement identified the process of how to actually conduct observation of patients for safety. In contrast, the RIE in the summer of 2011 was also focused on observation of patients. The differences in this one was not the basic safety focus, but now that we have improved overall safety of patient care, the focus has shifted to how we decrease this restrictive intervention and trust that the patients safety will not suffer. Physicians and nurses revealed their fears and concerns to improve patient care through more appropriate levels of observation. This clearly was the next or higher stage of culture change. This RIE was one of our most successful, both in producing the culture change of encouraging critical assessment when assigning types of observation orders as well as achieving our financial targets.

Lessons Learned

In the first 6 months of monitoring the metrics, a savings of more than $500,000 was realized in decreased numbers of patients on one-to-one observation.

Figure 7.6 illustrates the difference in dollars spent on 1:1 staffing during similar time periods before and after the RIE.

This is the type of patient care analysis we can expect to provide when our long-term goal is recognized as a true wellness and recovery model and center of excellence. We cannot raise the bar of practice without secure footing at every level. The basement of our structure is solid and complete. As we add another level, we must be mindful of the basic tenets that assisted us in achieving that solid foundation. We need to keep our feet in the gemba.

"Excellence Beyond Compliance" has developed as the mantra for the transformational change of the culture and climate for the KCHC Behavioral Health Service. Attitude adjustment, commitment to professional development, and a shared vision and practice of patient-centered care are needed to continue to complete this transformation. As we start measuring staff engagement and satisfaction,

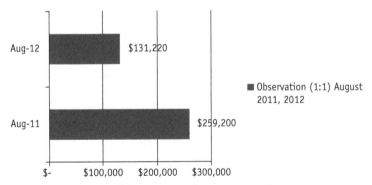

Figure 7.6 Financial impact of the Nursing Observation rapid improvement event: dollars spent on 1:1 staffing in the inpatient service during same time period in 2011 and 2012.

it is hoped and expected that the newly opened roads of communication, together with the higher bar of attaining excellence in patient care, will translate to improved staff satisfaction. Then we will know that we are truly on the road to excellence beyond compliance.

The new experiential knowledge gained through participation in lean activities and events has followed the participants back to their work areas, and they have stayed committed to working in teams for the benefit of our patients—beyond the scope of the lean event in which they were involved. They gained a new or enhanced sense of confidence in teamwork and, although difficult to measure, we feel this confidence brings a latent added value to the patient (our customer), to the organization, and to the community (our stakeholders).

The testimony we solicited from staff who participated in lean events (most of them for the first time) is rich with evidence of a sense of identity and investment in the success of the various products and processes they helped build and with a better understanding of the mission and vision of the department. A natural and welcome byproduct of staff engagement in lean events has been the recognition and appreciation for the value of teamwork. Staff from diverse backgrounds, with different educational, professional, organizational, and life experiences formed deeper relationships while working together on generating solutions to challenging problems. In conclusion, we faced a mandate to transform an inpatient service with just about every clinical process in need of reconstruction. We embarked on refocusing our services with regard for the patient's viewpoint, in alignment with the professional evolution evidenced in other areas of American medicine[2]. This major task required complex changes in clinical routines, better collaboration among disciplines, and changes in the organization of care.

Others have pointed out the multiple and often unpredictable interactions arising in particular contexts and settings that determine the success or failure while implementing changes[3]. Most of the available models and theories for the successful implementation of change are based on similar principles[4-7]. There seems to be wide agreement on the model for creating an implementation plan for change in health care[8]. Central to effective implementation is a systematic, well-planned approach that considers all relevant factors. This approach needs to use both the perspective of "the implementer" (the group wanting to achieve the change) and the perspective of the target group (professionals, team, service) receiving the proposal to change its performance. For the implementation to be successful, the entire target group must be committed to it. As far as possible, the target group should be involved in both the development of the innovation for change and the implementation plan[9]. We considered the "target group"—our staff buy-in—central to our success of implementing, and sustaining, change. The philosophy of lean—that the people doing the jobs are the ones who know the most about it, that a physician's opinion is no more or less important than that of the front-line nurse or orderly[10]—made it a natural choice given our identified priority of engaging our staff in true and lasting transformation.

Notes

1. Choi, T. (1998). The successes and failures of implementing continuous improvement programs. In Liker, J., *Becoming lean.* - Portland, OR: Productivity Press.
2. Laine, C., & Davidoff, F. (1996). Patient centered medicine. A professional evolution. *JAMA*, 275(2): 152–156.
3. Greenhalgh, T., Robert, G., Macfarlane, F., Bate, P., & Kyriakidou, O. (2004). Diffusion of innovations in service organizations: systematic review and recommendations. *The Milbank Quarterly*, 82(4): 581–629.
4. Bartholomew, L. K., Parcel, G. S., Kok, G., & Gottlieb, N.H. (2001). *Intervention mapping: Designing theory- and evidence-based health promotion programs.* Mayfield, CA: Mountain View.
5. Davis, D. A., & Vaisey, T. (1997). Translating guidelines into practice. A systematic review of theoretic concepts, pratical experience, and research evidence in the adoption of clinical practice guidelines. *CMAJ*, 157(4): 408–416.
6. Ferlie, E.B., & Shortell, S. M. (2001). Improving the quality of health care in the United Kingdom and the United States: A framework for change. *Milbank Quarterly*, 79(2): 281–315.
7. Green L. & Kreuter M. (1991) *Health promotion planning: An educational and environmental approach.* Mountain View, CA: Mayfield Publishing.
8. Wensing M, Wollersheim H & Grol R. (2006). Organizational interventions to implement improvements in patient care: a structured review of reviews. *Implement Science*, 1:2.
9. Grol R, Wensing M & Eccles M (2005). *Improving patient care* (pp. 290, 1st Edition). Oxford: Elsevier.
10. Suneja A. & Suneja C. (2010). *Lean doctors: A bold and practical guide to using lean principles to transform healthcare systems, one doctor at a time.* ASQ Quality Press Milwaukee, Wisconsin.

8

Outpatient Services

The Adult Mental Health Clinic

JILL BOWEN, LANCELOT DEYGOO,

AND TODD HIXSON

You have just read about the challenges of running an acute inpatient service; it is likewise a challenge to run a large psychiatric outpatient clinic, especially one that serves an inner city community with multiple complexities of need. The Kings County Hospital Center (KCHC) Behavioral Health Adult Outpatient Clinic serves central Brooklyn, a community comprised of a large number of immigrants, most of whom hail from the West Indies. The social challenges for new immigrants, plus the urban realities and social stressors, contribute to the demand for mental health service. There are many feeders into the adult ambulatory mental health clinic, which sees about 30,000 visits per year in this one clinic alone. These referral sources include the adult KCHC inpatient service, the Comprehensive Psychiatric Emergency Program (CPEP), medical services, and direct referrals from the community.

As described in previous chapters, the burning platform that erupted with the legal investigations focused on the acute care services (i.e., psychiatric emergency and inpatient services). Breakthrough events and application of lean methods were used in the KCHC CPEP and on the BH inpatient services to kick-start and support the dramatic and rapid transformation in those areas. Similarly to other hospitals in the Health and Hospitals Corporation (HHC), the scale of the Behavioral Health programs and their financial challenges provided enough rationale to mobilize major improvement initiatives, as can be seen in the before and after chart (see Table 8.1).

The ambulatory services were initially considered somewhat outside this flurry of activity occurring on the acute care services even though aftercare provisions in the United States Department of Justice (U.S. DOJ) settlement agreement required follow-up after discharge for 30, 60, or 90 days depending on the circumstances of

Table 8.1 **Summary of Adult Mental Health Clinic Improvements Using Lean**

	Before	After
Average Caseload	125	85
Average Billable Visits	1780	2452
Denials	210	95
Average Monthly Revenue	$100,349	$177,146

the patient. Nevertheless, the need to consider the whole continuum of care, while improving the performance of our organization, quickly became apparent. We were attempting to address the needs of the entire person and therefore could not comfortably fragment the work that was underway. Best practice models involving recovery and wellness principles were under development by the department as we moved to adopt a recovery-oriented philosophy of care. Recovery as a philosophy of care is a concept that emphasizes individual goals and outcomes and the impact of services provided in assisting people in meeting their goals. As noted by Sowers (2005), "Promotion of recovery has recently been recognized as an organizing principle for the transformation of behavioral health services." In his role as president of the American Association of Community Psychiatrists, Sowers presented the *Guidelines for Recovery Oriented Services* developed by the American Association of Community Psychiatrists.

Definitions of recovery tend to include hope and faith, self-management and autonomy, restoration and personal growth, dignity and self-respect, and peer support and community life, among others. These ideas led us naturally to look at our aftercare planning and community integration processes for those we served. According to the "Working Definition of Recovery from Mental Illness and Substance Use," Substance Abuse and Mental Health Services Administration (SAMHSA) delineated four major dimensions that support a life in recovery: health, home, purpose, and community. Recovery does not take the same form for every patient. It may include more traditional forms of treatment, including psychopharmacology and psychotherapy, as well as support from families, significant others, and stakeholders in the community, requiring a culturally sensitive workforce with a patient-centered approach.

An integral and crucial aspect of the U.S. DOJ Consent Decree for discharge and aftercare planning mandated that KCHC actively pursue the appropriate discharge of its patients in the most expeditious manner. This required KCHC to develop and implement many new practices and procedures to obtain compliance in this key section of the consent decree. It necessitated the creation of discharge and aftercare plans that would ensure that patients receive services in the most integrated and appropriate setting in which they could be reasonably accommodated. In addition,

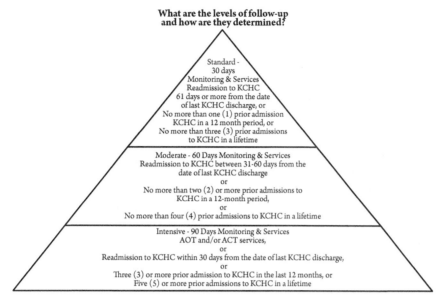

What are the levels of follow-up and how are they determined?

Standard -
30 days
Monitoring & Services
Readmission to KCHC
61 days or more from the date
of last KCHC discharge, or
No more than one (1) prior admission
KCHC in a 12 month period, or
No more than three (3) prior admissions
to KCHC in a lifetime

Moderate - 60 Days Monitoring & Services
Readmission to KCHC between 31-60 days from the
date of last KCHC discharge
or
No more than two (2) or more prior admissions to
KCHC in a 12-month period,
or
No more than four (4) prior admissions to KCHC in a lifetime

Intensive - 90 Days Monitoring & Services
AOT and/or ACT services,
or
Readmission to KCHC within 30 days from the date of last KCHC discharge,
or
Three (3) or more prior admission to KCHC in the last 12 months, or
Five (5) or more prior admissions to KCHC in a lifetime

Figure 8.1 Postdischarge follow-up—30-, 60-, 90-day criteria.

KCHC had to ensure that the discharge and aftercare plans were patient-driven, recovery-oriented, and created with the active participation of, and input from, the patient. KCHC was required to provide transition supports and services to adequately assist the patient in transitioning to the new setting, as well as ensuring continuity of care with appropriate community providers to minimize the risk of decompensation and reinstitutionalization. The DOJ requirement was to ensure that patients were discharged to, and integrated into, the most appropriate level of care. Although this approach was consistent with the recovery-oriented philosophy of care, the level of follow-up was beyond what had been typically expected, with no other acute care institution required to do this nationally to our knowledge. We were challenged to develop new approaches to achieve these new expectations for breadth and depth of postdischarge follow-up (see Figure 8.1).

Attention, therefore, moved from inpatient to outpatient care. Our focus on the clinic coincided with fiscal and regulatory changes in New York State, which added additional motivation to move our redesign efforts to the adult outpatient clinic.

In December 2008, the New York State Office of Mental Health (OMH), our licensing body, was telling us about an overhaul of the current system that was to take effect beginning March 2009. OMH undertook a multiyear initiative to restructure the way clinics were delivering services and how these mental health services were reimbursed. An advisory workgroup consisting of a broadly representative range of local government officials, mental health providers, and mental health advocates was formed. They were known as the Mental Health Clinic Restructuring Workgroup. This group was charged with advising OMH on ways to create a mental health system focused on recovery for adults and children and that would redefine clinic treatment services. In addition, attention would be paid to plans to restructure the financing of the mental health treatment system. Parallel to these changes the OMH recertification survey process was redesigned.

Restructuring the clinic seemed necessary to respond to the opportunities for enhanced services to patients and increased revenue that would accompany those changes. If properly poised with an infrastructure that could make use of them, then both clinical and fiscal opportunities could be maximized.

It was clear that the current system needed to be changed. Evolution of the outpatient mental health infrastructure was not new to New York. Over the past 50 years New York's mental health system moved from one dominated by the large state psychiatric hospitals to a dispersed system of nonprofit organizations, state, and private hospitals. There are currently more than 2,500 mental health programs providing Medicaid- and non-Medicaid-funded mental health outpatient, emergency, residential, community support, vocational, and inpatient services to more than 700,000 individuals annually. New York, like many states, expanded Medicaid funded mental health services. Today, Medicaid pays more than 50% of the more than $5 billion dollars annual cost of public mental health services. Even with this increase in Medicaid dollars, the system was not reflecting the changes in our service delivery model. As a result, there were several problems.

Outpatient services could not grow to meet expanding need because of the State's mental health neutrality policy. Half of the public mental health dollars financed psychiatric hospitalization. Reimbursement for clinic services was complex and inequitable. Short-term Medicaid initiatives such as COPS (Comprehensive Outpatient Program Services) programs, which provided some financial support, had become more like permanent solutions. Further, inadequate resources were devoted to early identification and treatment, despite recognition of their worth. There was also insufficient access to specialized services, including case management, vocational services, housing, employment, and children's waivers for those with extraordinary needs.

Many patients reported that the system seemed plagued with poor communication and a lack of accountability. Fragmentation, including poor coordination of services, limited integration between mental health and substance abuse services, as well as between mental health and physical health care was evident. It is well documented in the literature that those with serious mental health challenges often have high rates of medical comorbidities and often have poor health care habits and less-than-optimal medical care. Patients treated in our mental health services frequently did not follow up with medical appointments. Annual physical exams were not always completed or were not completed in a timely manner. Internists and psychiatrists did not confer regularly. This resulted in patients having their debilitating health conditions unaddressed or underaddressed. Medical issues such as obesity, diabetes, cigarette smoking, and hypertension were frequently present in the mental health population. There were concerns about potentially shortened life expectancy among those with mental health challenges, 25 years less on average, as well as high no-show rates for medical care. Federal regulations and continuous reinterpretation of approved state financing practices put the state, counties, and providers at substantial financial risk.

The Mental Health Clinic Restructuring Workgroup's task was based on the following guiding principles: clinic treatment should be a defined set of services (e.g., prescreening, assessment, therapy, medication management, medication administration); quality of care should include identification and engagement of clients; treatment services must be accessible to clients at clinics, off-site, and in the home; and phase out of the rate add-on systems, such as COPS programs.[6]

A change of particular interest to us, from both a clinical and fiscal perspective, was that the new system would allow for billing of multiple services provided the same day, using HIPAA-compliant billing codes. These codes are approved by the American Medical Association and meet a national standard for electronic health care transaction and national identifiers for providers, health insurance plans, and employers.

OMH's prior system allowed for reimbursement for only one service per consumer per day, with the exception of crisis and collateral services. The new payment methodology, to be implemented on the advice of the OMH Clinic Restructuring Workgroup, would be based on a new procedure-based (CPT) clinic reimbursement methodology. It would eliminate COPS payments, establish new peer group rates, and bill using CPT billing codes. The general rule was to provide payment by a "threshold" formula; for example, clients could have only one medical visit, one mental health visit, and one substance abuse service a day, and each service would be weighted against the established peer group rates, whereas before only one service provided could be billed per day. The result of the prior one visit per day billing plan was that either the patient had to return multiple times so the facility could capture payment for all services rendered (not very patient-centered), or the facility would provide the needed services on the day the patient visited and forego payment for many of the services delivered (not very facility friendly).

Now that we understood the playing field and had some sense of the new rules, we needed to transform clinic operations to maximize both the clinical and fiscal potential inherent in the new system. The specifics of the burning platform for the ambulatory clinic was thus multidetermined, including clinical, fiscal, and regulatory pressures for change. Knowing these changes would be taking effect soon, leadership was faced with the significant question of how best to proceed. As we prepared, we also had to address the fact that revenue collections were far from what we would have liked them to be and the clinic itself felt chaotic for both patients and staff.

We had to look at the current system with an eye to how to incorporate the new clinic restructuring regulations and opportunities in a manner that the clinicians could readily adopt. Mechanisms needed to be put into place to support the provision of multiple services on the same day, to reduce the need for clients to make multiple trips, to minimize missed appointments, and to enhance revenue while increasing patient satisfaction and adherence to their plan of treatment. We needed to maximize our billing opportunities, reduce denials, and streamline the financial clearance process. The savings that would be obtained through increased efficiencies and through improved customer service and processes was a vital focus of the overall lean approach.

The reasons for action were clear and the stage was set for us to do something big. The first rapid improvement event (RIE) for the mental health outpatient program at Kings County Hospital was planned.

In the current state, patients and staff experienced the environment in the clinic as disorganized and intense. It was not the atmosphere of choice for a therapeutic milieu. Some staff members described it as feeling like an emergency room. Patients would often show up at times other than their scheduled appointment, and there were intensive, well-meaning attempts to scramble to find the therapist or prescriber of record to meet with them. This made the reality of the daily work rather stressful, as these impromptu visits would need to occur between scheduled appointments. This attempt to meet on-demand requests led to unrealistic expectations. The reality of significant waiting time proved highly frustrating. Prescriber coverage felt stretched very thin, even for regularly scheduled appointments, with challenging attempts by the therapist to coordinate the medication management and therapy sessions. Rather than a clearly defined team model, a phase model (described below) had evolved. This phase model made for cumbersome patient flow and uneven caseload assignments. On the whole, caseloads felt quite overwhelming and ran rather high, although frequency and type of session varied by phase. This was not patient-friendly in that those who received services at the clinic would need to change therapists and prescribers as they moved into different phases of treatment, ironically disrupting the continuum of care while attempting to foster it. A need for a more organized, equitable, and therapeutic experience for those who received their treatment in the clinic, as well as a higher quality work environment for staff, was necessary.

The Phase system originally developed out of a need to increase access and decrease waiting time as visits increased. The New York City Department of Health and Mental Hygiene supported this initiative in 2007. Although initially this had some positive effect, flow and organization issues soon emerged. Phase I was designated as the "Early Recovery/Reintegration" Phase. In this phase, stabilization, extended evaluation, psycho-education, and empowerment occurred in a group setting. This allowed for the elimination of a waiting list, as all patients could quickly be incorporated into the group program. Patients were familiarized with the different services rendered at the clinic and the expectation for treatment adherence. This several-week phase ended with a disposition conference in which next steps for the patient were determined. Most patients went on to phase II, that of active treatment. This could be individual or group work. The staff had a difficult time transitioning from individual work to group work and difficulty absorbing the patients from phase I into phase II. The focus of the providers on individual work and the generally limited integration among various providers reflected the staff's holding on to an outdated private practice model. Phase I became longer and longer. Staff in phase II began to have caseloads that were too large for them to manage, with caseloads of approximately 120 for some of the clinicians.

Phase III was the maintenance and relapse prevention phase. In this phase patients attended monthly or quarterly groups or individual appointments aimed at maintaining their stability and the progress they had made during active treatment. Not all patients moved from phase I to phase II to phase III (some went from phase I directly to phase III), but most did. This sense of movement to an appropriate level of care within the clinic did not take into account the up and down nature of most mental illnesses. Recovery is nonlinear, characterized by continual growth and improved functioning that may involve setbacks. Because such setbacks are a natural, although not inevitable, part of the recovery process, it is essential to foster resilience during treatment approaches for all individuals and families.[7]

Staff were assigned by phase, and therefore, as patients moved between phases, they had to work on termination from one set of providers and re-initiate with another. This led to a current state in which staff often preferred to hold on to patients rather than moving them along to the next phase of care. This resulted in caseloads which were high but inconsistently so among the phases. Patients remained in phase II for far longer than their circumstances required. Rather than move to the appropriate level of care, phase II caseloads ballooned. Interdisciplinary work was loosely organized and each phase tried to manage their areas independently. The hoped-for continuum of care became a series of independently functioning silos with little integration into a system of continuous care. This was very "un-lean" in that it did not produce continuous flow.

Much needed to be reorganized to successfully transition to the new requirements and expectations. Preparing for the OMH restructuring meant reviewing the assessment, engagement/retention, communication, and risk processes; the development of safety plans; and the review of the large caseloads to assess which patients needed continued care. The new approach for survey reviews developed by OMH required risk assessments at intake and at least quarterly thereafter, along with treatment plan updates.

Communication among providers was to be closely reviewed to ensure proper supervision and hand-off. OMH designed their review around "anchors" that would be measured utilizing tracer methodology to follow the patient through their experiences in the clinic. If present, the anchors would be scored as either "adequate" or "exemplary." It became clear that the current state would not easily support successful recertification reviews or essential processes for optimum billing of services provided. Attempts to improve communication across phases highlighted their cumbersome nature and begged for a team organization that supported communication by its very structure.

Early attempts to address these difficulties between phases included the development of a templated note that would ensure that key information was passed from one treating clinician to the next as patients moved from one level of care in the clinic to another, but this proved insufficient and did not address the difficulties inherent in the phase system. The information included in the template note was helpful but did not allow for a full hand-off of information from provider to provider or for a more in-depth discussion with opportunity for questions to be asked and answered. Most importantly, it was insufficient to support the transition of the patient who would need to move to a new provider.

Transition to a new provider is challenging for patients and for staff, often involving separation of a therapist and provider where a working relationship had already been established. This disruption to the therapeutic process was not patient-centered and served the clinic's organizational phase structure rather than the patient. In addition to the disruption in treatment flow, the intake process itself was quite fragmented from the rest of the operation and integration was necessary there as well. It was also increasingly clear that the problem of equitable distribution of patients, and generally high caseloads needed to be tackled if quality of care was to be improved.

It was apparent that restructuring needed to take on the scheduling system, staff reassignment, delivery of care, and coding/billing to be in compliance and to maximize the opportunities inherent within the NYS OMH new clinic restructuring. Data for the previous year showed visits for the Adult Outpatient Clinic were less than would be expected. Essentially, the viability of the clinic was at stake—not only from a fiscal perspective but also from a regulatory and clinical perspective.

As we looked at the processes at play in the current state of the clinic, the waste and complexity involved in moving through the system became clearly evident. Visual management tools proved quite helpful in developing the target state. Steps in the patient flow and staff processes were outlined on the board and different colored and sizes of post-its were used, representing different types of steps. Lean helped us in understanding and delineating the difference between value-added and non value-added steps. For the clinic, value-added processes from a patient's perspective really boil down to receiving the treatment they need to get better, whether that is in the form of therapy, medication, or both. All other steps are essentially non-value-added as far as the patient is concerned. Certainly wait time, paperwork, and even insurance-related processes are non-value-added from a patient's perspective. Some of these steps may be necessary for other purposes, such as billing, but many are full of waste that can be reduced while enhancing the value-added aspects of the service the clinic provides. Stepping back and looking at the visual representations of the current versus the target state helped tremendously to show what is possible in this transformation.

During this outlining process of the work in the adult mental health clinic the multiple steps and the different people involved in the multiple steps emerged. The post-its representing different roles and steps helped to highlight duplicative and highly wasteful processes. It was no wonder the clinic felt chaotic.

A serious streamlining of operations was needed. This required us to review the forms that were used, in addition to the number of steps a patient needed to go through to get from intake to treatment (see Figure 8.2). Forms can be the bane of any clinic staff member's existence; staff will tell you that the work becomes the form rather than the form facilitating the work. This is a common problem; as forms are often developed to resolve particular problems, they tend to be added to, but never subtracted from. The more it became evident that complex processes were needed for adequate communication as patients moved between phases, the more the question was raised—do the patients really need to move from one clinician to another? Are the phases value added?

The target state was developed by first allowing the rapid improvement team members to imagine an ideal state. This opportunity to imagine the best possible clinic without the multitude of constraints that exist in the real world frees up the creative process. The target state, then, includes the basics of the ideal state: a clinic that runs smoothly, with excellent communication and clear expectations.

Standard work accomplishes a great deal in providing clear expectations for the entire staff. Standard work in a lean approach is one in which the details of a specific role are spelled out and represents the best known way at the time of accomplishing a task. Not only do people in different roles understand clearly the specifics of their responsibilities, but others in the clinic know this as well. Standard work once developed is then posted in the Gemba so all staff could refer to it as needed. Changes to the standard of work that become apparent over time are presented to the steering

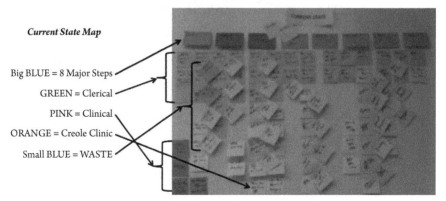

Figure 8.2 Rapid Improvement Event for Clinic Restructuring—Current State Map visually representing major steps in the operational process, highlighting waste.

committee for consideration and approval, and the changes made and posted. It is helpful to have all standard work dated. The target state for the clinic included the development of standard work for every role and task in the adult outpatient clinic. Duplication is thus removed and the logic of movement from intake to treatment team is preserved.

Streamlining of processes required a redesign of all the forms used, in addition to the roles of the clinic intake workers. This included every step in the process, from insurance verification to risk assessment to ongoing treatment and documentation. Accountability is difficult in a system with duplicative responsibilities and unclear roles. Once the processes and work for each staff member was standardized, the expectation of the target state would include accountability or ownership in the system.

The target state as visualized in the RIE included increased productivity and increased revenue. The target state metrics of 40,231 services/year reflected the new billing methodology of services and not visits and projected collections of $2,059,886/year. The data to be targeted included the number of visits, the amount of revenue collected, productivity by staff members, and their discipline (see Figure 8.3).

Now that the current state and target state were mapped out, the difference between them was obvious. The gulf between where we were and where we wanted

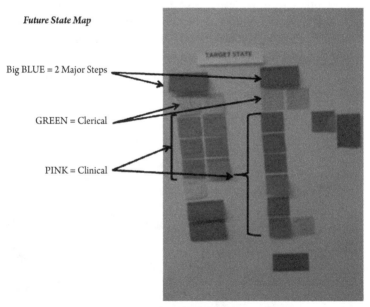

Figure 8.3 Rapid Improvement Event for Clinic Restructuring—Target State Map visually representing major steps in the operational process, plan for streamlined operations post RIE.

to be needed to be crossed. The gaps needed to be delineated and understood. The next step was to do just that: a gap analysis.

Gap Analysis

The gap analysis is an interesting process that helps move forward the work in understanding key barriers to success. By utilizing a process of trying to understand the root causes of the identified problems, as opposed to just addressing the surface problem, solutions can be identified that have a greater chance of making lasting and sustained change. In the clinic, these key areas were identified as giant caseloads, unnecessary paperwork, staff (as in the right staff doing the right job), reorganization of space, and Kings County Hospital attitude or culture.

GIANT CASELOADS

The average caseload at the time of the outpatient reorganization RIE was 125 patients per clinician. Although unevenly distributed, the large caseloads made the staff feel overwhelmed and weighed down by the responsibility of being on top of that large a number of ill patients. Although the frequency of seeing the patients varied from one or more times a week to quarterly, and unevenly by phase, the overall number was negatively impacting the morale of the staff and their ability to function well. Using the "five whys" process to keep pushing deeper to understand the root cause of the problem, staff first identified that there was difficulty in making discharge plans for patients. Teams focus on key gaps and seek to determine meaningful solutions through root cause analysis. Like curious children, participants in this analysis do not accept wasteful practices or other gaps as self-evident but endeavor through repeated questioning (why?, but why?, etc.) to delve more deeply into underlying causes to derive solutions with greater, longer lasting impact.

A challenge for many clinics working with patients who have serious mental illnesses and complex presentations is that post-clinic treatment options are often quite limited. Integration is also an important challenge in the development of recovery-oriented services, including substance abuse and mental health co-occurring disorders and mental health and medical comorbidities, suggesting the need to develop alternatives for the provision of care of mental health patients.[8] An open front door and a closed back door clearly lead to problems of large caseloads and long waiting lists. As the "whys" continued to be explored, the staff identified the problem of lack of sufficient discharge plans for patients. Looking deeper at this problem, they identified as a major area of concern the limits of outside resources, as well as the lack of a clear strategy to link to those outside resources, as seen in Figure 8.4.

Table 8.2 **Five Whys Approach to Understanding Root Cause**

What?	Why?	Why?	Why?	Why?	Why?
GIANT CASELOADS	No discharge plans for patient	No outside resources identified nor any strategy to link to resources	No dedicated staff with specific skills to assist with discharge	Not built into the program	Not part of the culture of the clinic
UNNECESSARY PAPERWORK	Lack of planning over time for the big picture	Regulations are complicated and changing	We are not completing the forms and not in compliance and so more forms are created	Staff caught in the middle and always behind in the paperwork	Lack of pruning and purging of forms
STAFF (right staff doing the right stuff)	Lack of planning, training, and team approach	Clinic was ignored due to CPEP and Inpatient issues	OPD leadership not heard	BHS in survival mode and neglected OPD	BHS was neglected by KCHC, HHC, and SOMH
REORGANIZATION OF SPACE	Lack of informed planning-staff levels increased and original plan note amended	Staff not involved in planning-never enough space	Leadership did not consult with OPD staff	It's the culture not to consult with staff (but maybe there was nothing they could do)	Leadership and staff are not communicating
KCHC ATTITUDE	Lack of accountability to patients and staff	"Just a job"; staff are apathetic	Low expectations; No incentives	No recognition of good work; No standards; Not customer satisfaction-based	Staff and patients not valued

IRL

Information, Referral & Linkage

- Work with patients/families in negotiating systems within the hospital and in the community
- Provide information about community and governmental resources.
- Assist with the implementation of aftercare plans including providing referral, linkage and advocacy services.
- Escort recipients into the community and make home visits as needed.
- Work closely with related social service and community agencies

RARC

Repeat Admission Review Coordinator

(Supervises the MRL's)

MRLU

Monitoring, Referral & Linkage Unit

Ensuring that patient's individual needs are met in the community, including need for housing, treatment, support, medication, public benefits & recovery

Figure 8.4 Components of the Community Linkage Unit.

This problem in the Kings County Hospital Behavioral Health Department as a whole was beginning to be addressed via a Linkage Unit focused on improving connections with community resources. This initiative developed as the acute care services struggled with the need to enhance connections with community providers as they looked to expand aftercare planning options. The OPD clinic saw an opportunity to learn from what had already been developed in the department, adapt and adopt those processes, and integrate them across the continuum of care. Lean emphasizes the importance of complementing data with direct observations in the gemba or specific workplace. Teams visited the clinic repeatedly to understand actual administrative and clinical practices and to see and document firsthand where excess steps and handoffs, variability, or poorly organized work areas contributed to defects, delays, and other forms of waste.

Process mapping and charting also proved quite useful. Step-by-step workflows revealed points of multiple handoffs, batch processing, and unbalanced effort. Teams prepared process maps of both initial and target conditions and itemized gaps between them to organize problem issues into such categories as process, policy, people (e.g., skills and knowledge), or plant (e.g., space and equipment) for further analysis. Teams also documented wasted time and motion by tracing excess patient and staff movement on floor plans and by charting information transfers on hand-off circles.

As the RIE team dug deeper into the root cause of the giant caseloads, they identified that there were no dedicated staff in the clinic with the specific skills necessary to assist with discharge and the linkages necessary to assist people with moving to the next level of care. This skill set had not been built into the program, they concluded, because it was not considered part of the culture of the clinic. Mental health clinics do tend to accept, more or less, that a large percentage of the patients they serve will need to remain as clinic patients for the foreseeable future. This has led to access limitations at many clinics, as expansion is often not a realistic option. Also, such a belief system is not consistent with a recovery philosophy.

UNNECESSARY PAPERWORK

Working through the root cause of unnecessary and excessive paperwork led to an understanding that insufficient time was set aside for completing required paperwork. Because regulations can be complicated and change over time, the staff came to the understanding that incomplete forms led to poor regulatory compliance, which ultimately led to more forms being created. This vicious cycle left the staff feeling stuck in the middle and always relentlessly behind in their paperwork. Taking the five whys all the way through, the final understanding of the cause of unnecessary paperwork was felt to result from a lack of pruning and purging of forms. With the OMH restructuring underway the time was right for a forms re-do from top to bottom.

STAFF (RIGHT STAFF DOING THE RIGHT JOB)

The question was raised: Were the right people in the right jobs; was there a good match of skill set to responsibilities? This is a centrally important theme in the transformation of any system and was addressed repeatedly as work progressed across the continuum of care. Interestingly, in the work to redesign the outpatient clinic, it was felt that the root cause of staff mismatch had a good deal to do with lack of planning, lack of training, and lack of a team approach. Digging further into the whys of this phenomenon, it became apparent that the staff felt the clinic as a whole had been ignored while the acute care services struggled with the challenges of responding to the DOJ investigation, settlement agreements, increased scrutiny, and intensive efforts toward transformation in those areas. The staff felt that clinic leadership's expressions of concern were not heard because of the overall feeling of behavioral health being in survival mode. The clinic staff had felt neglected. Now it was their time to put to use the methodology that lean had brought to bear in the acute care services.

REORGANIZATION OF SPACE

Although the clinic, along with the majority of the Behavioral Health Service, moved into a new building which was designed several years earlier, in February 2009 they quickly felt constrained by the lack of space for their increasing needs.

The crux of the five whys exploration led to a sense of insufficient line staff involvement in the planning of space for the new clinic. The root cause in this case was reflective of an overall sense of the need to improve communication, particularly between leadership and line staff. This was felt to be an issue of operations culture. Leadership and staff were not communicating optimally.

KINGS COUNTY HOSPITAL CENTER ATTITUDE

The KCHC attitude was described as, essentially, a morale issue. The five whys revealed a sense of a lack of accountability to patients and staff, who feel the work is "just a job" and have a general sense of apathy. The root cause analysis here uncovered low expectations and a lack of incentives. Good work was not felt to be recognized; it seemed that there were no clear standards and that the focus was not on patient satisfaction. The ultimate root cause was described as the lack of value placed on both patients and staff in the clinic setting.

The gap analysis laid bare key areas that blocked the clinic from improving performance in significant ways, which contributed to a less than satisfactory experience for both staff and patients, and blocked the staff from achieving target levels on the variables identified as necessary for viability and success. The solution approach enabled the group to look at the gaps and apply an "if we," "then we," approach to closing them (see Figure 8.5).

This methodology allows the team to lay out their ideas and consider actions and their likely results. For example, in looking at the giant caseloads and feelings of chaos, it was stated, "If we streamline intake process and have six treatment teams... Then we can create flow in the clinic and radically reduce caseloads!"

A major thrust of the redesign was identified clearly as needing to move from a phase system to a team system. This would address the large caseloads as well as the flow problem for patients as their treatment requirements changed. Redesign was to be rapid and clinic-wide. Within 30 days the three phases were to transform into six teams. Each team was to have a psychiatrist or psychiatric nurse practitioner (to perform assessments and medication management), a nurse (for health and medication education), social worker and/or psychologist (as primary therapists), and a case manager (to help with discharges). Including line staff in this redesign process was clearly necessary as the previous lack of inclusion in planning was an identified root cause to not achieving success in the clinic. The lack of planning, training, and team approach identified in the gap analysis would also be addressed by involving the staff in the development of standard work for all disciplines and all roles.

The solution approach put a great deal of emphasis on inclusion and communication among all levels of the clinic staff. Collaboration was clearly highlighted as essential to the sustainability of the improvement efforts. Bringing order to the chaos that was experienced in the clinic would come from the creation and implementation of standards of work, as well as a streamlined intake process that would

Gap:	If We:	Then We:
Current stat PHASE System of Treatment creates giant caseloads and lack of flow:	If we implement RIE design in 2 stages....STAGE 1: Re-assign staff from 3 Phases to create 6 Teams; Form discharge & outreach team; Create process to transition patients; Review current cases for appropriate level of care and disposition...	Then we can execute complete redesign within 30 days of RIE!
Lack of structure leads to feeling of chaos of patients and staff	If we streamline intake process and have 6 treatment teams...	Then we can create flow in clinic and radically reduce caseloads!
Lack of planning, training and team approach	If we involve staff in the planning, development of standard work, provide training and hold staff and leadership accountable...	Then we add value to the OPD experience; increase collaboration and sustainability of OPD improvement efforts
Leadership & staff not communicating	If we use Breakthrough tools & RIE redesign plan as a road map...	Then we improve morale which will improve patient care which will improve treatment environment

Figure 8.5 Solution Approach to addressing gaps between current and target states.

create flow in the clinic and hold staff and leadership accountable. The six teams and the improved flow would be designed to greatly reduce caseloads and ultimately provide the environment necessary to achieve the target metrics, including increased visits, revenue, and decreased denials.

Rapid Experiments

Lean transformation is intensive. The Behavioral Health Services as a whole was undergoing rapid improvement. One of the key methods that helped to ensure that efforts were directed appropriately and usefully were the rapid experiments that took place during the RIEs (see Figure 8.6). This allowed for course correction and modifications to the plan that was being developed during the week of the RIE event.

INSURANCE VERIFICATION SYSTEM

To ensure that the intake process that was designed to decrease waste, increase patient flow, and decrease the sense of chaos in the clinic was on the right track, a rapid experiment was conducted to determine if the use of a new insurance verification system (state Medicaid verification terminal) would work as intended. We connected a State Medicaid verification terminal, and we ran the patient Medicaid insurance card before the patient was seen by the clinician. This system is designed to enable clinics to verify, in real time, if the patient's insurance is active and the type of insurance they have (i.e., Medicaid fee for service or Medicaid managed care) and whether this insurance is within our network. If the patient had Medicaid managed care insurance, then their information could immediately be referred to a managed care coordinator and authorization for the visit obtained. The results confirmed that the approach was a good one and four additional machines were to be ordered.

Experiment:	Expected Results:	Actual Results:
Install a pilot EMEV machine in OPD area	More detailed insurance verification system	1 installed—detailed insurance verification! 4 EMEV machines ordered!
Reduce and streamline various OPD forms	Develop a user-friendly product to enhance flow	Produced good working DRAFT of streamlined forms to pilot!
Flow data through new staffing pattern design	Improved flow and development better team structure	New staffing pattern with better flow that reduce caseloads
Explore new treatment algorithm to inform treatment planning	Consultation with HHC Central Office regarding progress of algorithm	Obtained working draft of HHC Central Office algorithm; partnership agreed to complete!

Figure 8.6 Rapid Experiments to test solution approaches.

STREAMLINED FORMS

Good working drafts of streamlined forms were also developed and given a test run during the rapid experiment phase. The user-friendly forms showed much promise in enhancing patient flow. The new staffing pattern made sense as they practiced the flow of the data through a six-team structure versus a three-phase structure. The rapid experiments validated that the plan designed was ready to move forward.

Completion Plan

The completion plan is where much of the work that has been designed and tested is put into effect. This is not an easy process as it involves training, follow-through, and commitment to maintain the momentum generated during the RIE event. Items on the completion plan typically need to be addressed within a month's time if at all possible. The completion plan for the clinic included quick fixes, known as "just do its," which would move things forward quickly toward achieving the goals. These included items such as installing insurance verification machines and phones with dedicated lines with outside access for intakes. An office was to be dedicated for nursing examinations. New forms needed to be reviewed and approved through appropriate processes.

The completion plan also included processes that were not "just do its" but could be accomplished within 30 days. Most significantly, the completion plan included staff reassignment from the three phases to the six teams. In addition to changing the organization of the team structure, the patients needed to be transitioned to their new teams. To achieve this task cases needed to be reviewed and appropriate level of care and disposition determined. In addition to the formation of the treatment teams, a discharge and outreach team was to be created. The case reviews included determining which cases remained active cases and which would need to be transferred to new therapists. Those staff who were a part of the phase III stabilization team would receive active treatment cases of patients who required more frequent sessions. Those who had been members of phase II would have some of their caseload switched to include stable patients who required only quarterly sessions. The caseloads would thus be distributed more equally and fairly, and patients would be able to stay with their treating therapists and prescribers regardless of level of care needed in the clinic. Every attempt was made to minimize disruption to our patients, our customers for whom we were endeavoring to add value to the services they were purchasing from us.

The discharge and outreach team would work with the treatment teams to focus on postclinic planning and to increase the options in the community. The members of this team were to be linkage specialists who would coordinate with the Linkage Unit that had been created for Behavioral Health as a whole. The treatment teams would now be poised to respond to the requirements of the OMH restructuring, including improved interdisciplinary treatment planning and communication, risk assessment, and safety planning.

A key component to a completion plan is the training necessary to bring all staff onto the same page. Standards of work, new forms, new flow processes, and team formations needed training and support for successful implementation. Clinic leadership, with support from BH leadership, would spearhead the effort at training, but it was the clinic members of the RIE that would prove most critical to achieving buy-in from the rest of the clinic staff.

Confirmed State

The confirmed state looks at the metrics to be measured, their baseline rate, and target. For the clinic redesign, demand in terms of visits was an essential metric. OMH redesign would enable increased services per visit, an opportunity for improved integration of care as well as increased revenue. Quality metrics, including productivity, would also be affected and would work hand-in-hand with increased services. The improved team approach would make it much easier to coordinate various services, while decreasing chaos and uncertainty regarding services rendered for patients, as well as for staff. Revenue metrics would then reflect the increased visits and services, as well as the increased productivity of the clinic staff.

Steering Committee Review

Every month the behavioral health executive steering committee meets to go over the breakthrough events that are open and to discuss upcoming breakthrough events. In reviewing the clinic restructuring event we found that productivity and collections were increasing but the standard of work was encountering a few problems with scheduling, coding, and billing, and although we saw an improvement, it was not enough to prepare us for the changes that would be coming with the new OMH clinic restructuring. In March 2010 we were told by OMH that the clinic restructuring that was scheduled to take effect in March was being pushed back to July 2010. This gave us some time to revisit any problems we were having and expand on the success of the RIE that had been done.

The Behavioral Health steering committee thought it would be beneficial to add an additional RIE for the Adult Mental Health Clinic, with the realization that one such event was insufficient for the scope of changes necessary for this program. Another rapid improvement event was scheduled in April 2010, to focus more specifically on scheduling, coding, and billing in the adult outpatient clinic.

Clinic Rapid Improvement Event #2

The Adult Mental Health Clinic was still encountering problems with scheduling appointments for clinicians, financial clearance, and insurance verification for potential and current patients as well as coding and billing for services rendered in the central intake unit and other clinical areas. The previous Adult Mental Health clinic RIE had a standard of work for the clinic but it became clear that greater specificity was needed when it came to the support staff duties. The current state did not have templates in the scheduling system for every clinician; there was no centralized appointment system leading to no checks and balances. This led to decreased numbers in productivity for clinicians and lost revenue opportunities.

We wanted to centralize the appointment system and put forward a detailed specific standard of work for scheduling patients. A standard of work to address the steps to be taken for a screening for insurance verification and appropriate financial clearance was also needed, as was a standard of work to address coding and billing for visits and services provided in the clinic.

In the Gap Analysis we found that a training for staff in the use and capabilities of the schedule program was needed. We needed to give the support staff access to the scheduling program but needed an identified staff member to work with the clinicians in maintaining their patients' appointments in the clinic. Scheduling and communication between clinicians and support staff were not centralized. Responsibilities and roles for these activities were not clearly defined.

The new "R" building is the home of our outpatient clinics and our adult mental health programs. A design feature of the new building was the co-location of inpatient services on the same floors as outpatient services in the hope of enhancing aftercare treatment adherence. It was identified that two financial counselors covering the many programs in the building was insufficient. Our support staff was overwhelmed resulting in a negative impact on our bottom line.

The two financial counselors were located on the ground floor of the "R" building and patients from nine outpatient programs were referred to them by the registration staff. Some patients were not following through with a visit to see the financial counselors because of the distance between the location of the financial counselors and the location of the clinics. This was not patient-centered as it required a patient to move from the outpatient program on the upper floors to the finance area on the first floor and back upstairs again to the outpatient program. We therefore relocated the financial counselors so they could work side by side with the registration staff in the outpatient programs. This move was critical in ensuring we saw all patients for financial clearance and insurance verification at the point of registration.

This RIE also identified that communication between support staff, clinicians, and finance was limited and data to inform the current problems was not readily available. We needed to ensure that ongoing training would be given to the support staff to ensure that improved communication between clinicians and support staff would be achieved. Greater access to the current system for all eligible staff was identified as essential. A detailed standard of work needed to be created for the support staff to ensure all roles and responsibilities would be clearly defined. Collaboration with Information Technology was identified as necessary to look at the current scheduling system and to upgrade or address any deficiencies. Accomplishing these changes would address the lack of access and knowledge that was present at both management and staff levels, which impacted productivity, patient care, and staff turnover. Once accomplished, this would ensure that the scheduling system would be utilized effectively.

We looked to do several rapid experiments immediately. We opened up templates in the Unity Scheduling system and experimented with 15-minute slots, explored overbooking and documenting no-shows. We found that the templates which existed could be modified to allow for scheduling in 15-minute slots and for overbooking. We looked at the Emev insurance verification system as compared with an alternative system, the hospital HFE, and determined that although both were working efficiently the Emev, Medicaid web-based application used to check insurance information in real time, had the edge for us. It provided a means for verification that could be attached on the encounter form to show it was done via tape print-outs.

Work began in earnest on the completion plan. All clinician schedules had to be filled out first on paper for review and subsequently entered into the electronic scheduling system. Schedule templates had to be built for all clinicians. Support staff needed to be trained in the new standard of work and in scheduling and insurance verification.

Additional steps taken to accommodate the OMH clinic restructuring included designing our own encounter form, which utilized visual management support by displaying insurance information that was in-network on one side of the form, to help the registration clerks quickly and easily identify the correct insurance. This was very helpful to the support staff and the form doubled, efficiently, as a reporting tool for the gathering of necessary information. The other side of the encounter form showed the individual services available for billing and the next scheduled appointment. This encounter form covered all of the requirements highlighted in the two outpatient mental health RIE events. Also implemented was a reconciliation system to ensure we were billing for every service and visit provided and a system to clear every scheduled patient financially before their visit.

Improvements don't always take effect immediately, and some of the anticipated results following an RIE do not come to fruition as quickly or precisely as one would hope. That was true for us as well in the adult clinic. Caseloads, for example, did not immediately shrink upon the completion of the first RIE for the adult clinic, although that was a key component of that event. Over time, however, with the second RIE and continued adherence to standard of work, the caseloads did show a steady decline (see Figure 8.7).

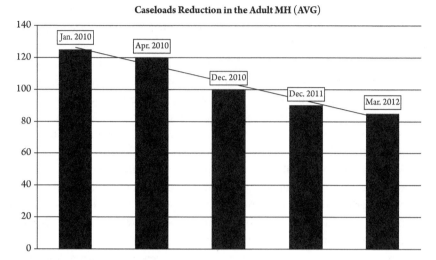

Figure 8.7 Caseload comparison from January 2010 through March 2012.

Sustainment

The RIE that led to successful redesign of the outpatient clinic was the first of several events over the course of the next year and a half for the adult clinic. The redesign took place at the end of January 2010, and the subsequent event described briefly above regarding scheduling, coding, and billing took place in April 2010. In June 2011, an RIE was held to work on interservice integration as the work on flow through the continuum of care expanded to include movement from inpatient services to outpatient services. This was a successful attempt to remove unnecessary steps in the outpatient admission process for those who were discharged from our own inpatient services. No-show rates were decreased by removing the intake step and allowing for direct admissions from adult inpatient to adult outpatient services. Data showing sustainment in increased revenue, visits, services, and decreased denials has been continually tracked. This is a notable and sizable impact on the adult outpatient clinic operation in a rather short period of time, with clear and meaningful outcomes. Lean enabled this transformation, bringing improvements in organization, accountability, coordination, and communication.

It should be noted that the state OMH clinic restructuring took effect in October 2010 and we were ready. Payment for services on a phase-in process did not take effect until January 2012, retroactive to October 2010.

As of February 2012, we had an increase in billable visits, from 1,780 on average per month to 2,452 on average per month, a 36% increase over baseline (see Figure 8.8).

Our denial rate also dropped over this period, reflecting a 55% decrease in denials over baseline (see Figure 8.9).

Adult Mental Health Clinic
Average Billable Visits

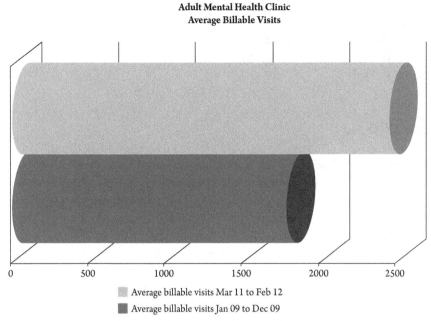

Average billable visits Mar 11 to Feb 12
Average billable visits Jan 09 to Dec 09

Figure 8.8　Increase in average billable visits before and after RIE.

Adult Mental Health Clinic
Average Monthly Denials

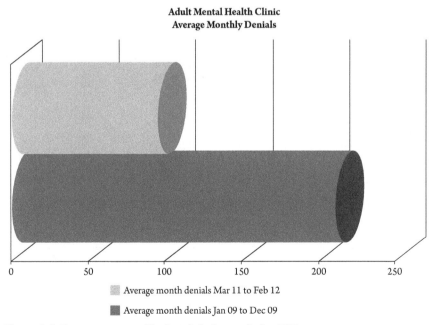

Average month denials Mar 11 to Feb 12
Average month denials Jan 09 to Dec 09

Figure 8.9　Decrease in monthly denials before and after RIE.

For services per visit, by February 2012, 42% of average monthly visits included more than one service during a visit (see Figure 8.10).

And finally, and most gratifyingly, overall revenue increased to an average of $177,146 /month over the baseline of $100,349/month, a 76% increase (see Figure 8.11).

Insights

Lean in behavioral health was initially focused on improving acute psychiatric care at the inpatient and emergency room level. Nevertheless, outpatient goals evolved as behavioral health leaders grew more comfortable with lean methods and more open to challenging longstanding problems and as it was realized that the entire continuum of care needed transformation.

Performance does not quickly improve in clinical programs where operations and practices developed over years are entrenched and accepted by the staff as the way things are done. In this environment, fundamental and sustained change is possible only when staff members begin to see their work differently and transform their thinking, and that transformation is only possible after repeated cycles or waves of improvement activity using the same process and perspective, as is the case with lean.

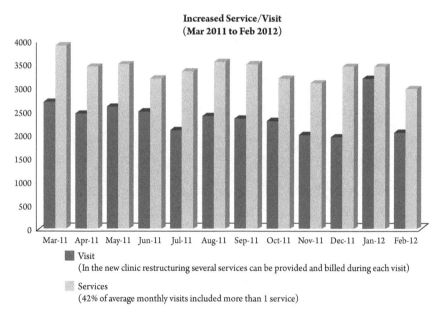

Figure 8.10 Utilization of multiple services per visit in the Adult Outpatient Clinic.

Adult Mental Health Clinic
Average Monthly Revenue

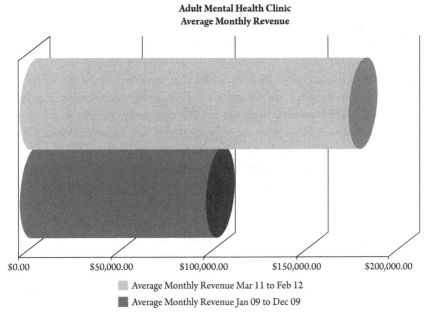

| $0.00 | $50,000.00 | $100,000.00 | $150,000.00 | $200,000.00 |

Average Monthly Revenue Mar 11 to Feb 12
Average Monthly Revenue Jan 09 to Dec 09

Figure 8.11 Increased average monthly revenue before and after RIE.

Historically, results from individual interventions may be incremental at best and elusive at worst, but gains accumulate rapidly as staff revisit their problems and processes and gain the deeper insights and solutions that result. Work around solutions are revealed as ineffective band-aids if metrics are faithfully monitored and changes that seemed radical or impossible at first become increasingly acceptable, even necessary, as cycles of improvement continue.

Lessons Learned

Business processes were easier to change than clinical processes and practices. Because improvements in encounter reporting, patient registration and the like relieve annoying paperwork burdens and burnish managers' financial results, most staff embrace them, if only after the fact. By contrast, interventions in the clinical milieu can threaten physicians' and therapists' notions of their independence and clinical judgment and initial resistance can ensue. Nevertheless, a continuous focus on the improvement efforts needed to address barriers to patient care, and on the influence that disconnected or seemingly unrelated processes have on clinical outcomes and workloads, eventually leads most clinicians to accept change, if grudgingly at first.

Going forward with the subsequent VSA and our new round of RIEs, there was acknowledgement of the need to follow up on the achievements in the clinic and focus on the work that still needed to be addressed there. These areas of focus include important next steps in improving quality and flow in the clinics and include: admission and discharge criteria for the outpatient clinics, the integration of ambulatory medical care, the integration of partial hospitalization into the service flow, the referral process from inpatient to outpatient and expansion of group work in the clinics. These events promise to bring significant improvement to the outpatient operation and bring the clinics further along the lean journey alongside its acute care counterparts. All part of the incremental daily improvements in quality.

Those who have participated directly in the lean events are enthused and motivated by the experience. They take ownership for their event and work hard to bring the new approaches to the areas in which they work. In looking over the course of events in the clinical chapters of this book it becomes evident that increasing the participation of staff at all levels of the department is crucial. Further, utilizing lean approaches is more than a series of RIEs. Rather, it is an approach to problem solving that is inclusive, data-driven, and provides clear expectations of roles which allows for improved accountability. A3 thinking, utilizing the nine boxes of an A3 design organizes thinking into the areas delineated in the clinical chapters of this book (Reason for Action, Current State, Target State, Gap Analysis, Solution Plan, Rapid Experiments, Completion Plan, and Insights). Once the lean approach is understood and becomes integrated into the day-to-day operation of an organization, the A3 approach becomes broadly useful with multiple applications, which sustains improvements and supports transformation at all levels and across all services in the department.

Staff Insights

- "Everyone in [the] hierarchy can contribute to process."
- "Functions of different areas and support from management brings Change."
- "Taking care of one area makes participants want to take care of others."
- "Although some of us have worked in the department for years, we learned more about group therapy this week than ever."
- "Helpful to see new direction of Psychiatry and everyone's part in it."
- "Good vehicle for change to break down barriers and territoriality."
- "Better way to see deficiencies and need for connections."
- "Clinic redesign will increase the safety net for our patients."
- "Our goals are ambitious but attainable."

This is particularly important in behavioral healthcare today in which complex realities of managing multiple services and integrating both the traditional continuum of care along with medical and mental health care, substance abuse, and mental health issues, and community integration pose significant challenges. The evolving landscape of regulatory, fiscal, and best practices requires managers and clinicians to be prepared with tools to meet these changes head on and continue to provide the vital services for the patients and the communities we serve.

The process of participating as a member of a rapid improvement event is often a powerful and empowering one. Below are voices of the internal customer, descriptions of their experiences, and their insights following participation in lean event.

Notes

1. Adams, N. & Grieder, D.M. *Treatment Planning for Person-Centered Care. The Road to Mental Health and Addiction Recovery.* Elsevier Academic Press, 2005. pp. xx–xi MA, USA.
2. Sowers, Wesley. *Transforming Systems of Care: The American Association of Community Psychiatrists Guidelines for Recovery Oriented Services,* Community Mental Health Journal. Vol. 41, No. 6, December 2005. Pp. 759.
3. SAMHSA: Working Definition of Recovery from Mental Illness and Substance Use, http://www.samhsa.gov/recovery/, March 23, 2012. Accessed August 7, 2013.
4. www.omh.state.ny.us/omhweb/clinic_restructuring/report.pdf *Clinic Restructuring Inplementation plan.* Office of Mental Health, March 11, 2009. Accessed August 7, 2013.
5. Corrigan, P.W., et al. *Principles and Practice of Psychiatric Rehabilitation.* The Guilford Press, 2008. pp. 346–358. New York: Guilford Press.
6. OMH op.cit.
7. SAMHSA op. cit.
8. Sowers op. cit.

9

Lean Applications

The Medical Home Model

CLAIRE PATTERSON, JANINE PERAZZO, AND AKINOLA ADEBISI

With rapidly changing mandates in health care, the Health and Hospitals Corporation (HHC) is facing a number of practical challenges to improving the safety and quality of patient care while making that care more affordable. This chapter will explore the ways in which the organization is moving toward delivering seamless, high-quality, patient-centered care in an environment where the patient and providers are true partners in care decisions.

In early September 2013, HHC received designation to participate in the Medicare Shared Savings program as an Accountable Care Organization (ACO) from the Centers for Medicare and Medicaid Services (CMS). The designation formalizes a new type of relationship with HHC's existing physician affiliate partners: the Physician Affiliate Group of New York, the New York University School of Medicine, and the Mount Sinai School of Medicine. These three entities employ virtually all the physicians working in HHC hospitals.

The Medicare Shared Savings program is part of the federal Affordable Care Act and is geared toward decreasing health care spending by preventing unnecessary emergency department visits and hospitalizations for Medicare patients who receive the majority of their primary care from providers associated with the ACO. The premise of the program is that with a combination of robust primary care, better care coordination, and more effective care management will result in healthier patients at a lower cost. Qualified organizations have an opportunity to share in the resulting savings.

HHC has worked hard in recent years to create patient-centered medical homes and Health Homes, to improve patient care through adherence to evidence-based protocols, and to improve patient health through more effective chronic disease management. Collectively, this work is intended to benefit the patients and communities served, and all of it is very relevant to our ultimate success as an ACO.

As a large, integrated health care delivery system, our construct positions us well to provide the seamless, patient-centered, coordinated care expected under the ACO program. Succeeding as an ACO will represent a significant step toward our strategic goal of achieving better care at lower costs without compromising our mission: to serve all New Yorkers, regardless of their ability to pay. It will also put us at the forefront of health care reform, positioning us for the similar shared savings opportunities New York State is exploring for parts of the Medicaid population.

So what does it mean to transition to an ACO, and how does it relate to much of the work we are already doing to improve patient care and increase efficiency in Behavioral Health Service at Kings County Hospital Center (KCHC)?

The March 2012 Value Stream Analysis (VSA) provided the impetus for the Behavioral Health Services (BHS) leadership to sharpen our focus on deploying lean to support the strategic goal of closing the gaps in related activities to prepare us for the anticipated ACO designation. As we used lean to strip waste from our processes and improve care delivery, patient recidivism was at an all-time low and KCHC was one of the first HHC facilities to co-locate primary care and behavioral health care and offer enhanced services. Despite significant improvements, the system was still difficult for our patients to navigate, in part because not all of components of the care management model required for our Health Home designation were fully operational.

To ensure the gains from previous improvement efforts are sustained, to close remaining gaps, and meet the Triple[1] Aim (improve health, improve care, and reduce cost of care) for the Health Home program, BHS leveraged lean tools and techniques to achieve the target state as defined by the core clinical features for behavioral Health Homes:

- Each patient must have a comprehensive care plan.
- Services must be quality driven, cost effective, culturally appropriate, person/family centered, and evidence based.
- Services must include prevention and health promotion, health care, mental health and substance use, and long-term care services as well as linkages to community supports and resources.
- Service delivery must involve continuing care strategies, including care management, care coordination, and transitional care from the hospital to the community.
- Health Home providers do not need to provide all required services themselves but must ensure the availability and coordination of the full array of services.
- Providers must be able to use health information technology (HIT) to facilitate the work of the Health Home and establish quality improvement efforts.[2]

In this chapter we will focus on two rapid improvement events (RIEs). In the first, we introduced the concept of patient-centered care into the BHS Wellness and Recovery program. In the second, we improved access to outpatient care by effectively coordinating and linking members of the care team during admission and discharge processes.

Wellness and Recovery Rapid Improvement Effort

The Division of Wellness, Recovery, and Community Integration of KCHC BHS is responsible for identifying gaps in knowledge, understanding, and application of wellness and recovery principles among staff and other key stakeholders. This is accomplished by assessing education and training needs against the scope of the Recovery Model, including but not limited to recovery concepts, the Eight Domains of Wellness (see later discussion), psychiatric rehabilitation concepts, person-centered care, and emerging best practices, which are documented in experimental accounts of consumers and family members, literature from the field, and related theoretical frameworks. These concepts are discussed in more detail later in this chapter.

The complicated and challenging task of integrating this philosophy and these principles throughout the service of behavioral health is critically important to the transformation of BHS into a Center of Excellence that substantially improves patient outcomes and contributes to the advancement of the field. During the week of May 20 to 25, 2012, 11 staff members from across several disciplines and a patient/peer counselor participated on a Breakthrough (RIE) team that focused on just that. The team developed a communication plan titled "Everything Communicates Wellness and Recovery, Verbally, Vocally, and Visually."

WHAT IS WELLNESS?

The RIE team was charged with first establishing working definitions for wellness and recovery. Based on the established paradigm developed by Peggy Swarbrick and funded by SAMHSA, wellness is the successful interrelationship of diverse life domains and their impact on each other.[3] In layman's terms, this means that individuals are able to balance every aspect of their life in a way that is meaningful and fulfilling to them. The eight domains of wellness include physical, emotional, financial, environmental, occupational, social, intellectual, and spiritual dimensions.

WHAT IS RECOVERY?

Similar to wellness, there are numerous definitions of recovery, ranging from those posted by the traditional medical, to the academic, experiential, grassroots, social, spiritual, or other paradigms. However, the RIE team developed the following working definition:

> Behavioral Health Recovery is an individual journey of change which fosters the ability to adapt to one's personal experiences and to live a meaningful life in a community of one's choice.

To ascertain the current state of wellness and recovery thinking in behavioral health, the team surveyed both staff and peers regarding their perception of how recovery oriented the environment was in terms of images, treatment, and milieu.

After analyzing the current state, the interdisciplinary team (guided by our in-house Sensei, coached by our facilitator, and kept to task by our team leader) brainstormed for potential direct causes of the identified gaps. To narrow the enormity of the task, they focused on five key areas and targeted their interventions toward integrating recovery and wellness principles into thinking and practice. The areas for improvement were identified as follows (see Figure 9.1):

1. The Structure of the Wellness and Recovery Department, which was reorganized and is now called the Department of Wellness, Recovery, and Community Integration
2. Dissemination of expertise
3. Staff training
4. Recipient of care education
5. Monitoring and Continuous Quality Improvement (CQI)

In addition to the pillars of focus for wellness and recovery just listed, the team produced a drawing of the target state and drafted a position guidance paper as well (see Figure 9.1 and Box 9.1).

Basic didactic and informational training on the principles of wellness and recovery has been done service-wide since 2009, yet these gaps remained. Thus, the team decided a more advanced approach was essential, starting with the identification of three primary mechanisms for integration: (1) education and training, (2) coaching, and (3) wellness rounds and reviews. The following specific programs within the organization were identified as being successful at integrating the input of "recovery experts":

- Treatment team coaching
- Repeat Admissions Review Committee (RARC)
- Behavioral Support Team (BST)
- Critical education
- Core orientation
- Role of the peer counselor as recovery expert, "Ambassador of Empathy"

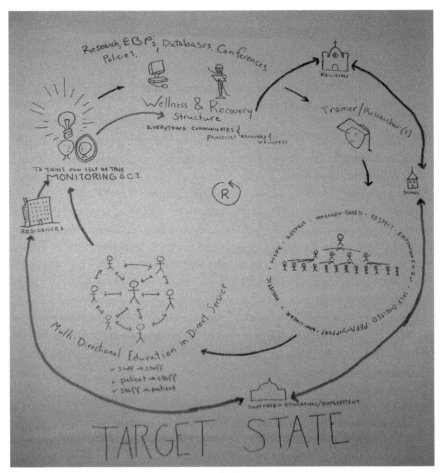

Figure 9.1 Rapid Improvement Event Team Members' Pictorial Depiction of the Targeted State for Wellness and Recovery at Kings County Hospital Center

The success of these education mechanisms is being measured by an assessment of knowledge, understanding, and application of wellness and recovery principles. This includes documentation of the use of recovery language in treatment team meetings, dialogue between individuals, and clinical documentation as well as evaluation of the methods of engagement utilized by the clinical teams. BHS has also implemented a monthly Recipient Perception Survey and a Staff Perception Survey to measure and collect data on utilizing the three recovery principles of hope, respect, and holistic care in treatment.

The impact of this RIE continues to evolve, and it is just one of many BHS initiatives that support our medical home deliverables. BHS is now able to more effectively utilize the data that are being collected in its efforts to advance integration of the wellness and recovery philosophy of care.

Box 9.1 **Position and guidance paper on structure and philosophy for wellness and recovery at Kings County Hospital Center.**

Position and Guidance Paper on Structure and Philosophy
Division of Wellness, Recovery, and Community Integration

Outline

I. Message on Transformation

    a. Systems –Healthcare Reform and National Policy on Behavioral Health

    b. Organizational ~ Video on Accountability Model, Mr. Aviles

    c. Community–Addressing Needs through Cultural Competence and Trauma~ informed Care

    d. Individual–Paradigm Shift: Treatment by Attraction, not Promotion

II. Philosophy of Care

    a. Recovery Principles

    b. Definitions & Applications

    c. Balancing Regulatory Mandates with Philosophy of Care

III. Division of Wellness, Recovery, & Community Integration: Fundamental Structure and Critical Componetns

    a. Restructuring of Department

        • *Experts*

        • *Supervisory Structure (W & R Staff; Peer Counseling Staff)*

    b. Staffing and Expertise

    c. Systems transformation

        • *Operationalization of Recovery Principles*

        • *Adopting Recovery~Based Language*

    d. Methodologies for Integration

        • Infusing Recovery~Oriented Care

        • Standards of Work

        • Training Models (reciprocal on~Unit Education; Staff Training, didactic, in vivo, observational, supervision, peer reviewed)

    e. Monitoring and continuous Improvement

        • Data~informed feedback to guide continuous improvement

        • Competency Assessment

        • LOS and Strategies for Empowerment and Person~Centeredness~Reassess Criteria for Involuntary Admission

        • Recipient Rights, Well~Being, and Satisfaction

IV. Appendices

    a. Resources

        • Wellness Plans

        • Advance Directives

    b. Bibliography

    c. Policies and Procedures

Box 9.2 **Behavioral Health Services Outpatient Department Admission Flow Chart for Patient Accessing Care From the Centralized Intake Unit**

```
┌─────────────────────────────────┐
│             CIU                 │
└─────────────────────────────────┘
        │
┌──────────────────────┐
│ All patients         │
│ recorded in          │
│ Registration Book    │
└──────────────────────┘
        │
┌──────────────────────┐
│ Walk-in patients     │
│ given data sheet to  │
│ completed            │
└──────────────────────┘
        │
┌──────────────────────┐
│ Pre-screen by RN     │
│ and determined       │
│ eligible for         │
│ assessment           │
└──────────────────────┘
        │
     ◇ Is patient          YES    ┌──────────────────────┐
       acute-danger  ─────────────▶│ Patient escorted     │
       to self?                    │ to CPEP              │
        │ NO                       └──────────────────────┘
        │
     ◇ Is currently in     YES    ┌──────────────────────┐
       treatment?  ────────────────▶│ Redirected patient and│
        │ NO                       │ explain importance   │
        │                          │ of continuity with   │
        │                          │ current treatment    │
        │                          │ team.                │
        │                          └──────────────────────┘
     ◇ If insurance        YES    ┌──────────────────────┐
       not accepted ────────────────▶│ Register patient and │
       by HHC                      │ patient will be seen.│
        │ NO                       └──────────────────────┘
        │
┌──────────────────────┐
│ Explain to patient   │
│ their insurance in   │
│ not accepted by      │
│ HHC and redirect     │
│ to participating     │
│ facility             │
└──────────────────────┘
        │
┌──────────────────────┐
│ Refer patient to     │
│ Case Manager or      │
│ Peer Counselor       │
│ for follow-up        │
└──────────────────────┘
```

The wellness and recovery approach extends well beyond the inpatient setting and has also taken root in the Outpatient Department (OPD) and in the Behavioral Health Primary Care Clinic, weaving elements of the pillars of focus into the linkages for continuity of care.

Outpatient Department Rapid Improvement Events

ADMISSION AND DISCHARGE RAPID IMPROVEMENT EVENT

To further improve workflows, additional RIEs were chartered for the OPD. The admission and discharge RIE was a crucial exercise for the outpatient clinic. There was unprecedented enthusiasm regarding this event as the theme was initiated from the "grassroots," a basic lean principle. Even prior to charting the course of the VSA, there were many concerns raised by the clinic staff regarding the significant problems of patient flow in the clinic.

In a public hospital psychiatric clinic, the imbalance between supply and demand creates many challenges. Kings County Adult Outpatient Psychiatric Service is the largest outpatient psychiatric provider in Central Brooklyn, with more than 2,200 active cases, and it has more than its fair share of challenges. The clinic is situated in a mid-to-low socioeconomic, predominantly minority catchment area, with many immigrant or first generation American-born patients.

In addition to chronic unemployment, many of our patients are undocumented, thus rendering them ineligible for government aid, including food stamps and Medicaid. This exacerbates psychological and physical consequences of poor nutrition and lack of access to timely medical care, which interact with the recognized factors of family instability, community and domestic violence, poor schools, substance abuse, and low self-esteem that often follow poverty.

As discussed in Chapter 8, there have been three prior RIEs held in the adult OPD. The Outpatient Department Redesign RIE held in Jan 2010 looked to transform our dated private practice model to a more modern approach to outpatient treatment in a clinic setting. The OPD Resource and Financial Integration RIE in April 2010 looked at the payment structure, and in December 2011 the "Intake and Discharge Flow Cell" noted some improvements in admission, treatment, and discharge processes but recognized significant duplicative practices that negatively impact the delivery of care.

The most recent RIE was held in August 2012 on admission and discharge criteria and aimed to develop the standard work for discharging patients to primary care. The standard work included refining criteria for admission to OPD, creation of guidelines for redirecting recipients of care (ROC) to the most appropriate treatment setting, improving access to care in the OPD, and an attempt to balance the marked unevenness of caseloads between therapists.

When one takes a step back to look at the nature of the RIEs over time, it becomes apparent that there has been a slow evolution in the actual content of the events. There has been a move from more "structural" or "nuts-and-bolts" issues (such as making sure bills are generated for services rendered, basic oversight, and supervision to ensure patients are being seen) to more "process-oriented" RIEs that focus more on the flow of patients, staff, and information. In essence we are now looking to make the existing systems more efficient, further reducing waste, another key lean principle.

It is noteworthy that on the surface, the topics dealt with in each event appear similar, with each new event working on fine-tuning the procedures developed from prior events. This reflects the reality of the ongoing work required to implement cultural change and Kings County Behavioral Health's goal of continuous improvement.

CHALLENGES AND TEACHING MOMENTS FOR OUTPATIENT DEPARTMENT

One of the first challenges of the most recent RIE was trying to select an effective multidisciplinary team that would work together efficiently. The adult OPD has only been involved in a fraction of the large number of events that have taken place in the CPEP and inpatient settings. Additionally, one of the objectives of the VSA—a 2.5-day event that takes the corporate, facility, and departmental goals and synthesizes them (i.e., lean's principle of alignment) into the themes of the events that will be carried out in the department each year—is to increase the total number of staff exposed to lean in a "hands-on" manner. The ideal solution was to create a team that included both veterans and novices to lean.

Two to three months before the event, the clinic leadership began brainstorming about the composition of the team. This is recommended by lean: Prework begins 3 months before the start date of your event. The choice of team leader was difficult. We considered several psychiatrists and social work supervisors but decided on a nurse practitioner with more than 2.5 decades of experience in KCHC, starting out as a registered nurse and completing her advanced training while working full time. She brought a wealth of experience from seeing the clinic through multiple transitions as well as a steady, low-key interpersonal style. The fact that she is currently studying for her doctorate degree also indicates her focus and determination. A prerequisite for the position is green certification (a basic level of lean competency achieved by successfully participating in a 1-day training), which was satisfied by the nurse practitioner's willingness to attend the corporate training and certification before the event.

The clinic leadership met alone and with our high-energy, free-thinking lean facilitator to begin to decide on the actual focus of the event and wrote their thoughts on the "leaves" of an "idea tree." Brainstorming was often facilitated through the use of these trees, which consisted of large, simply drawn trees with yellow post-its for

> **Lessons Learned**
>
> We recognized that recycling the same individuals who had been involved in prior RIEs would defeat the goal of increasing the overall staff numbers involved in the process. Organizations using lean need to be on alert for falling into the pattern of identifying a group of high-performing individuals who recognize the value of lean, and simply using the same or a similar cohort of individuals for all subsequent events. Having said this, it is also important to develop individuals to become more expert and to function as "embedded facilitators" within your value stream. Doing this will wean you from dependence on outside consultants and Sensei and will further spread lean throughout your organization. In the end it was decided that the new multidisciplinary team would consist of dedicated staff that had the potential of working well in a team but had no prior lean experience.

leaves strategically placed around the clinic so that staff could anonymously offer suggestions for the focus of an event. These tactics, as well as staff polls, helped ensure that the defined scope of the event incorporated all significant associated issues.

In a clinic of its size and with the various changing demands from payers, regulators, and the public, the temptation is to try to cure all ills and tackle more than can realistically be addressed in a single RIE. We had to be careful to clearly define the scope of the each event and exclude issues and categories that would best be managed by other events.

One of the foundations of lean work is having good data. The team was challenged by the lean facilitator until eventually we obtained data that helped us to set priorities for the event. Some of the data flew in the face of "accepted" general knowledge. For example, the team learned that out of a caseload of 2,100 patients, 45% carried diagnoses in the schizophrenia spectrum and more than 17% of patients carried diagnoses in the bipolar disorder spectrum. There had been an initial belief that at least 50% of the patients suffered from less severe disorders like anxiety and depression. Another misperception corrected with data was the belief that 50% of patients missed their initial intake appointments, contributing to a huge amount of waste. We found that for the period observed, almost 80% of initial appointments were actually kept.

Although great progress was made in previous RIEs in reducing average caseloads, we noted that the variation in primary therapists' caseloads remained unacceptable, ranging from 80 to more than 120 patients per therapist. An overburdened clinician is unlikely to provide optimal care, runs the risk of burnout and resignation, and is unlikely to be able to proactively reduce his or her caseload. We realized that the sheer volume of patients in the behavioral health clinic was a significant determinant of caseload size and variation between therapists. We decided to run another RIE, with this one focusing first on making it easier for behavioral health patients who could appropriately be treated in a primary care setting (where basic medication management could be provided) to be discharged successfully to the primary care clinic. This work reduced the wait time in the primary care clinic between initial intake and completion of the clinic admission process, and reduced the patient load in the behavioral health clinic sufficiently so that we could attempt to rebalance the caseloads of our clinicians.

During the event it was noted that one of the team members was carrying the highest number of inactive patients (patients not seen within 30 days of the last appointment). The team member was naturally resistant to exploring this at first but then admitted that completing the discharge process was not the highest priority and the paperwork involved took too long. A rapid experiment was conducted during the RIE to determine how long it would take to discharge patients. He completed the discharge paperwork in less than 10 minutes—less than half the time the team member felt it would take. The team member had a personal "breakthrough" experience in recognizing the value of the lean techniques and becoming more committed to the rapid improvement event, and consequently gained a more personal stake in the clinic's success.

Other rapid experiments showed that following a pathway algorithm would enable patients to be referred to an alternate level of care. Also, 18 of 23 patients who were identified as transferrable to the primary care clinic were indeed transferred. Other patients were identified as having completed treatment or as having the potential to be best served elsewhere, and the team was able to locate community resources in certain cases to transfer patients to.

One significant development from the event was improving the experience for patients who receive long-acting antipsychotic injections—this is a crucial and at times life-changing treatment for patients with chronic psychotic disorders who, resulting, in part, from suboptimal adherence to their medication regimen, have often experienced multiple hospitalizations. Once some of these patients began taking the long-acting forms of medication injection every 2 to 4 weeks, they experienced improved medication adherence without the worry of daily or twice daily pill regimens. For some patients, this begins the process of recovery without disruptive symptoms or the demoralization that accompanies repeated hospitalizations. They are now able to move forward in their recovery journey using therapy, social support, and time to heal.

Previously, patients receiving long-acting medications were required to see the psychiatrist or nurse practitioner on the fourth or fifth floor of the Behavioral Health building, notify the front desk clerk, go to the first floor to get the injection, and return to the clinic floors to hand over the encounter forms needed for billing and obtain a card for their next appointment and a public transportation voucher, if eligible, for their next visit to the clinic before the appointment was over. After reviewing the patient flow process and "spaghetti diagrams" (which show how often and how far people or equipment move in the process of completing a task), we decided that if the patient dropped off the encounter form required for billing in a folder maintained by the injection nurse, all forms could be picked up at the end of the day by finance personnel.

This would save the patient a second trip to the fourth or fifth floor, simplifying the process and saving the patient's time. This demonstrates the elegantly "simple" ways that lean development of standard work can reduce waste and improve efficiency while improving the patient's experience and fostering increased treatment adherence.

A second minor but significant development was electronically sharing initial appointment information with the Medical Records department and the psychiatrist or nurse practitioner the day before the appointment. Previously this information was only given to the therapist who would see the patient. By providing this information to Medical Records earlier, the chart could be available for the therapist to review the patient's history before the day of the appointment. Also, the psychiatrist and therapist would be able to coordinate their schedules and, preferably, both see the patient on the same day. This change enabled a more comprehensive and efficient assessment in fewer visits.

The new process also accrued financial benefits to the clinic as New York State's new insurance payment system gives clinics the incentive to provide multiple services on the same visit and penalizes providers that surpass specific thresholds of number of visits per patient per year. This, too, enhances patient satisfaction with the delivery of their care.

An experimental plan was added to give clinicians the option of pulling a patient from a pool of waiting patients in the event of a no-show. Although there are obstacles that may make fully implementing this adjustment to standard work impractical, it is demonstrative of an effort to maximize staff capacity while trying not to overburden them.

At the end of the event, targets were set to:

- Increase percentage of patients receiving an intake appointment in OPD within 30 days.
- Rebalance the therapist caseload in line with state guideline of less than 100 patients/therapist.
- Increase the number of patients who receive an appointment within 30 days of psychiatric evaluation in our intake area.
- Increase referrals/OPD discharges to primary care.

The flow chart algorithms shown in Boxes 9.2 through 9.8 were created to provide a guideline to assist with determining the best disposition and referral of patients in a variety of challenging situations. It was posted on all three floors of the clinic.

Staff Insights

"We worked well as a team." "Efficient work happens in numbers." "It was great to get to know my colleagues better." "Good progress with respect to discharging patients for OPD to primary care clinic." "At a loss for words! Amazing how many seemingly unnecessary steps are used to complete the process. Lean measures definitely needed."

"There are so many complicated situations that make a streamlined process difficult." "An amazing week, today with experiments, goals were met, great team work." "What an experience! Hope our good work is put into place soon."

What follows are some of the comments from members of the RIE team after they completed the week's work.

Some team members were inspired to write about their RIE experience. These include the following:

> The most positive experience for me was spending a large amount of time working collaboratively with my coworkers. The nature of our work in the OPD is often solitary, and little of our work is side by side with our coworkers on common problems. When we do collaborate it is often rushed and for short spurts of time during the day. By spending long periods of time together we were able to express more sides of our personality and build up more trust and stronger bonds.

> My RIE experience was a very good one. I felt invested in the outcomes, as I had an input. I felt valued in that our ideas and suggestions were really appreciated by administrative staff and our process owner. My team worked well together and was very cooperative. My experience gave me a different perspective returning to the clinic. Like an "awakening: and I felt rejuvenated. Since my return I have been approaching things like referral to BH-primary care differently with my patients and am in the process of referring two patients. I think everyone should have the benefit of an RIE experience at least once; it is eye opening.

At this point, our new standards of work are being rolled out to the staff. We are very excited about the process, and although we cannot predict the future, we do feel confident that the event will make significant improvements to the care we provide to patients and to the work environment of our dedicated clinical and clerical staff.

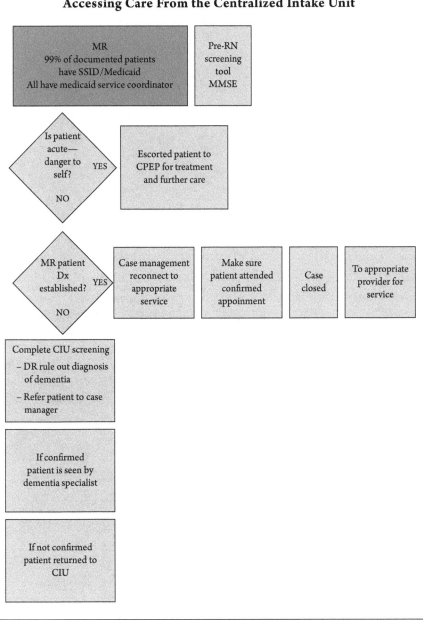

Box 9.3 **Behavioral Health Services Outpatient Department Admission Flow Chart for Patient With Mental Retardation Accessing Care From the Centralized Intake Unit**

MR
99% of documented patients
have SSID/Medicaid
All have medicaid service coordinator

Pre-RN
screening
tool
MMSE

Is patient acute— danger to self?   YES

NO

Escorted patient to CPEP for treatment and further care

MR patient Dx established?   YES

NO

Case management reconnect to appropriate service

Make sure patient attended confirmed appoinment

Case closed

To appropriate provider for service

Complete CIU screening
– DR rule out diagnosis of dementia
– Refer patient to case manager

If confirmed patient is seen by dementia specialist

If not confirmed patient returned to CIU

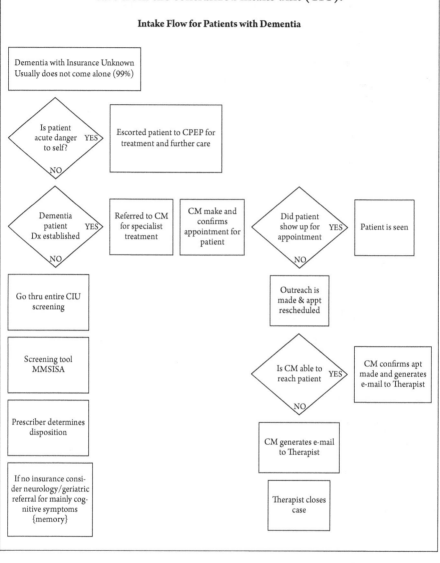

Box 9.4 **Behavioral Health Services Outpatient Department admission flow chart for patient with dementia accessing care from the centralized intake unit (CIU).**

Intake Flow for Patients with Dementia

Box 9.5 **Behavioral Health Services Outpatient Department admission flow chart for patient with substance abuse as primary diagnosis accessing care from the centralized intake unit (CIU).**

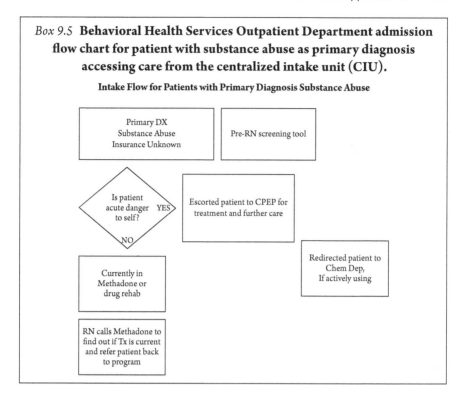

Intake Flow for Patients with Primary Diagnosis Substance Abuse

THE OUTPATIENT DEPARTMENT CLINIC HAS TWO MORE RAPID IMPROVEMENT EVENTS SCHEDULED FOR CURRENT YEAR

Integration of Care: Linkage to Primary Care and Establishing Ongoing Coordination of Care

Targeted areas of improvement include the following:

Establish and fully implement guidelines and a standard of work to ensure:

- Every outpatient has an up-to-date physical examination on entry to the OPD clinic and an annual physical exam thereafter.
- All medical needs are monitored and there is consistent communication between the outpatient clinic and medical providers.
- OPD patients will be linked to comprehensive and integrated ambulatory services that address their individual needs. (Improved referral and linkage with community mental health specialty care for more complex cases.)
- Easy access to mental health treatment for people with other serious or chronic illnesses, such as diabetes or cardiac conditions, whose recovery is impaired by co-occurring mental health disorders.

Box 9.6 **Behavioral Health Services Outpatient Department admission flow chart for patient requiring a higher level of care but refusing to be redirected based on his insurance coverage plan guidelines.**

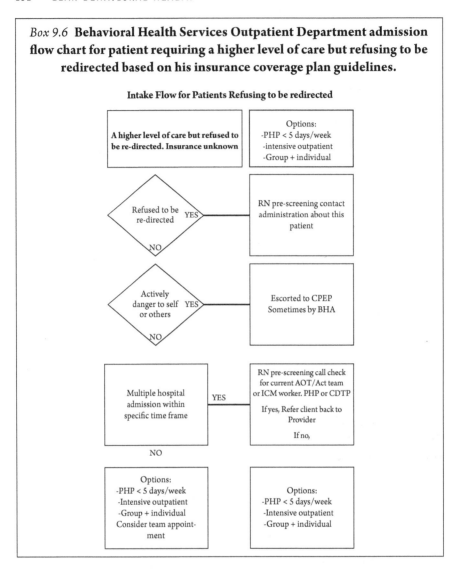

Linking Metabolic Screening to Primary Care

This RIE redefines the role of the OPD psychiatrist to require consideration of the whole person and assume responsibility for coordination of care among specialists, increasingly defining the role of a provider as one that integrates medical and mental health care.

Targeted areas of improvement include the following:

• Consistent monitoring of everyone on medication(laser focus: patients on Clozapine [Clozaril] and Olanzapine [Zyprexa] for metabolic changes).

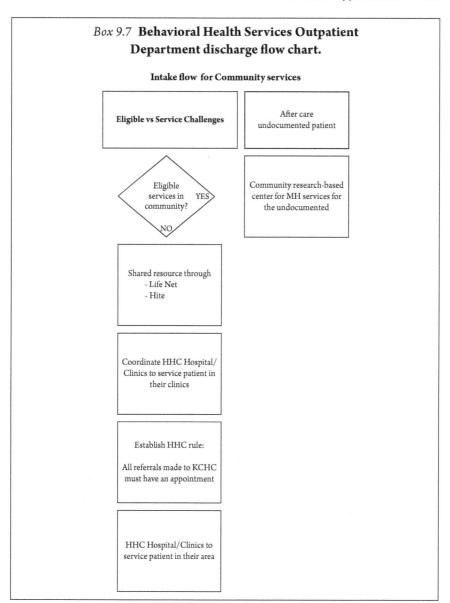

Box 9.7 **Behavioral Health Services Outpatient Department discharge flow chart.**

Intake flow for Community services

- If abnormalities related to the pharmacotherapy are identified, then develop a standard to coordinate referral and ongoing coordination with primary care to:
  - avoid onset of diabetes
  - improve monitoring of hemoglobin A1C for diabetic patients
  - improve monitoring of hypertension
  - improve monitoring of hyperlipidemia
  - improve monitoring of obesity

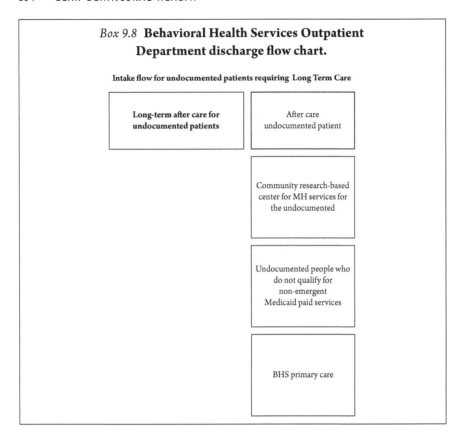

Box 9.8 **Behavioral Health Services Outpatient Department discharge flow chart.**

Intake flow for undocumented patients requiring Long Term Care

Long-term after care for undocumented patients	After care undocumented patient
	Community research-based center for MH services for the undocumented
	Undocumented people who do not qualify for non-emergent Medicaid paid services
	BHS primary care

We initially saw this as a lot of extra work—which it is! However, the more we use lean, the more we recognize that it is a tool to assist us in reaching our goals and not an imposed burden. We recognize that uncertainty and flux are the only predictable forecasts on the horizon for health care in the years to come. Lean, with its focus on continuous improvements, is certainly a steady rudder that can assist in guiding us through choppy waters and support our journey to building the ideal medical home model and becoming an ACO.

Notes

1. *Health Affairs*, May 2008; 27(3):759–769; doi: 10.1377/hlthaff.27.3.759. Accessed online August 5, 2013.
2. Centers for Medicare and Medicaid Services (November 16, 2010). Letter to state Medicaid directors and state health officials. Retrieved from https://www.cms.gov/smdl/downloads/SMD10024.pdf. Accessed May 15, 2013.
3. Swarbrick, P. 2011. *Defining Wellness,* http://welltacc.org. Accessed February 13, 2013.

Conclusion

JOSEPH P. MERLINO, JOANNA OMI, AND JILL BOWEN

We have shared with you our story of taking on the challenge of transforming a broken system—perhaps a somewhat unique story in the degree of change required and the scope seen in many behavioral health care settings. We believe that much of what we have learned will be informative for other behavioral health care providers, and many of the elements of our work are transferable to other behavioral health care settings. We began in a place of great challenge, with a burning platform that burned brighter than those of most organizations. The exercise of taking time to reflect on where we have been and how we have changed and been changed by our improvement system has been a gratifying experience. As never-ending day-to-day challenges compete for our attention, it is easy to forget or overlook the extent of the many positive changes we made to our behavioral health system at Kings County Hospital. Perspective and context are extremely useful, and documenting our efforts—both successful and not—for this book was an opportunity for us to pause, stand back, and see the big picture.

When our parent organization, the New York City Health and Hospitals Corporation (HHC), offered us lean as a means of addressing the complexity and urgency of our situation, it was not a system of change with which we were familiar. Nevertheless it was a system of change, and change was what was sorely needed in our hospital.

Lean is not a panacea, nor is it the only transformational approach available. However, some system to guide us was necessary. We were offered a technique and an opportunity. We were persuaded that we should try lean because at its core was a methodology that engaged staff at all levels in the process of identifying problems, researching solutions, and implementing corrective mechanisms—quickly! In other words, lean could help us bring about the culture change that was essential to fixing a very broken system.

In the insights we have incorporated at different points throughout this book, we have attempted to convey, at a personal level and in their own words, the experience of different people in our organization and the impact this approach has had on them. Understanding and listening to the voice of the customer, including those staff who are tasked with direct care, is a key to success. Lean is an inclusive process and inclusivity helps an organization move from a top-down approach of management to a more participatory organization, where success, and how to get there, is owned at all levels of the organization. The total support of leadership to follow through with decisions that come out of these events is critical to establishing trust and brings value and meaningfulness to the work of all staff.

Lean is a data-dependent, outcomes-driven performance improvement approach; that in and of itself was a major culture change for us. Performance improvement is typically driven by quality assurance processes; lean enhances this, and we soon realized that lean was performance improvement. It is designed to enable us to take the best of what we know about traditional quality assurance and pump it up to hour-by-hour and daily improvement while engaging the entire department and attaining essential business goals. Our approach to the use of data when we started our transformation efforts was anemic in terms of using data to inform decision-making. Many of the data points that were needed had to be obtained through laborious hand-counting procedures. Building a data shop and the infrastructure to support it allowed for increasingly effective monitoring and measuring, trend analyses, and accuracy of information—no more "GIGO." Use of data to provide direct and timely feedback to teams and providers on their performance proved invaluable to our forward momentum. Although we initially struggled to build the data sets and to utilize them meaningfully, we have become much more sophisticated in the use of data, providing and using key clinical, operational, and aggregate data that is now available on our desktops and at our fingertips and is incorporated at all levels of our clinical and quality improvement work.

In this book we have focused on organizational, quality, fiscal, and clinical issues specific to behavioral health. We have described some of the obstacles that were before us and explained how we worked to surmount them; some were successes and some failures. Why did some events yield such strong results and others not? Why were we able to sustain some improvements over the years while others faded? These are questions that continue to motivate us to strive for answers using the lean approach of daily improvement. Successes, we discovered, were more likely to come from human-sized scopes of attack and when focus was sustained on a particular service to give sufficient time for change to take hold before jumping to "fix" another problem. CPEP, our first clinical area of attention, remained our main focus for some time before we moved our efforts to the inpatient division of our hospital. Several small but significant events were planned ranging from clinical flow to patient property. Each one was doable and each one fed the overall functioning of the service, building on previous successes. The inpatient service, a much larger service encompassing nine separate units, tended to have greater success when programs were started on individual units and then built upon and spread to other units. Pilot programs initiated in limited areas that were spread only after sufficient testing and learning were more successful and were more sustained than attempts to implement new improvements across the service as a whole in one fell swoop. As such, understanding the need for a phase I and a phase II in a particular area of focus led to greater integration of changes to daily operations. The outpatient department has seen some significant and sustained change to date but is far from complete. We continue to refine our efforts in our clinic and strive for improvements there as new challenges continue to present themselves. Learning from our previous experiences, the adult outpatient clinic is undergoing various lean events to continue the solidification of previous efforts while expanding on the integrative work that has already begun there.

We have discussed several rapid improvement events (RIEs) in this book as we traversed the continuum of care in behavioral health. A major key to success is understanding that the pre-event period and the post-event period are as important as the weeklong intensive event itself. In fact, the prep is critical to the success of the actual event. These two periods, which sandwich the event week at 3 months out from the event on either side, ensure that the event is productive. Baseline measures and questions about current state are answered and "reason for action" is confirmed during the prep period. The scope of the event is finalized with an eye toward ensuring that it is a reasonable scope for success and that you are not over-reaching or "trying to boil the ocean." On the post side, the critical steps to success include training and implementation of standard work, following through on the completion plans, and monitoring the outcome data employing countermeasures as necessary.

As we became more comfortable with RIEs, we learned to use the problem-solving tools of lean in our everyday approach to daily improvement efforts using project planning, A3 thinking activities, and mini-retreats (a few hours to a day) aimed at more localized problems and processes. We used these approaches to improve our service related to mental health court processes, enhance our data shop, develop a violence task force, establish a staff wellness initiative, and develop standards of work in several areas, continually working to involve as many staff as possible in lean activities—a necessary part of achieving lasting impact.

It is undoubtedly key that not only does the hospital leader visibly support lean at Kings County Hospital but the regional and corporate offices are similarly visible in their commitment to lean. Vested in a system-wide effort, we believe that the work we continue to do at Kings County has "stick" and can be replicated throughout HHC. At the enterprise level, work has begun to capture and evaluate our work in preparation for site-by-site gap analyses for just this purpose.

The opportunity that lean brought to our organization went beyond the "True North" metrics of quality, safety, timeliness, human development, finances, and growth. Lean has enabled us to begin the several-years process of culture change. We have not achieved a culture change that resembles an ideal state by any means, and many of our staff still feel a sense of disenfranchisement from the department and from the decision-making process, but significant improvements have occurred and activities designed to further engage our employees are well under way.

The transformation is dramatic at Kings County Hospital Behavioral Health Services. We have been able to rise from an atmosphere of tragedy and public scrutiny to an organization that is the model in several of our innovative programs. We now receive international visits to learn about our Peer Case Management Program, are highlighted by the New York State Office of Mental Health as the place to visit for those developing and enhancing CPEP programs, and have received excellent feedback from oversight agencies on the advancements we have made across our continuum of care. We have become an organization that is achieving its goals and one that many of our employees, patients, and the community are proud to call their own. We are continuing to develop as a lean organization, becoming gradually but notably more self-sufficient in our use of the tools and techniques to achieve ongoing improvements and to ensure sustainment of the advancements we have made. We hope our story and our book can help you and your behavioral health care organization, clinic, or practice achieve the daily improvements required to provide our patients and community the high-quality affordable care they need and deserve.

Epilogue

Insights of a Psychologist Turned Lean Facilitator

KRISTEN BAUMANN

A few months after I moved from being a process owner for change in the Comprehensive Psychiatric Emergency Program (CPEP) to a full-time lean facilitator, a colleague left a copy of a *Wall Street Journal* article on my desk. With the article was a note that in summary stated, "Why would a talented clinician and respected leader become a *LEAN* pusher?" I had been taking some heat from my fellow clinicians as an early adopter but this was a tough one. I was prepared to read yet another article about how lean had failed. However, after reading the article, I was not sure my colleague had read the entire article or understood it.

The article, "Where Process-Improvement Projects Go Wrong," started with strong wording: "Recent studies suggest 60% of all corporate Six Sigma and like-minded process improvement initiatives fail to yield the desired result." Shortly after this introduction, it became apparent the article was exploring process improvement programs in large companies over a 5-year period to gain insight into how and why so many fail. Although the methodology was never disclosed by the author, the findings are relevant to our recent experiences at Kings Court Health Center and may act as a guide for those seeking to avoid process improvement failure with or without a sensei or coach.

There were four major findings from the research in the article. First, "extended involvement" of an improvement expert was found to be required if teams were to remain motivated, continue learning, and maintain early wins. It was noted that if a full-time expert was cost prohibitive, then it was found to be just as successful to have one assigned part time to several teams over 1 to 2 years while training managers to eventually take over the "expert role." Second, the research found performance appraisals needed to be tied to the successful implementation of improvement projects. Without incentives to motivate better work practices, employees often regressed to old ways once the initial enthusiasm for process improvement initiatives died down. Third, process improvement teams were found to be optimal at six to nine members, and implementation should be less than 6 to 8 weeks after the work. The study found that the larger the teams the harder to build consensus. Further, it was noted that delays in the implementation led to increased risks of people and resources being diverted. Finally, it was uncovered that executives need to directly participate in improvement projects—not just "support" them. The hands-on approach by executives allowed real-time analysis of both successes and failures, more meaningful countermeasures, and ultimately which projects were worth continuing.[1]

As a clinician, administrator, and now lean coach for one of our sister Health and Hospitals Center (HHC) hospitals, I have witnessed the need for "leadership" at the heart of these efforts firsthand. The use of quotations around leadership is to indicate that there are numerous operational definitions of this single word.

Kings Court Health Center (KCHC) Behavioral Health Science demonstrated leadership needs in roles at multiple levels of the organization over the past 5 years. My role as leader in CPEP from 2008 to 2009 forced me and my team to dig deep and ensure we had a balanced approach to leadership and that we were able to sum up all the changes required into one vision that we could check on together. We started with three goals: safety for our patients and staff, quality care, and patient and employee satisfaction. When patients and emergency medical service (EMS) workers asked why CPEP seemed a bit different as we changed, we knew our experimentation with change was working. What did that look like? For our patients and EMS workers, it meant coordinated and timely triage and assessment early and within required time frames. For our staff it meant less frequent silent disagreements during huddles, frank and productive confrontation, and letting go of "that's how we have always done that" conversations.

We have shared an improvement system with you in this book and have illustrated how to implement such a system using lean. We may not have stressed enough that leadership must be shared at all levels of the organization to bring about sustained change. It must be noted that many front-line staff have not been asked to lead nor have they seen themselves as leaders in their organizations, which underscores the importance of "spread" within lean organizations whereby more and more line staff are involved in events, thereby becoming "owners" of the changes, invested in their sustainment.

The complicated environment of leading to support teams beginning this journey needs to be explored. The challenges chosen for discussion below are in keeping with those reviewed in the change management literature and reflect our 4 short lean years thus far. This list is focused on the early stages of lean leadership as a way of scoping this discussion.

Leadership development, characteristics of successful leaders, and analysis of different management styles can be found in scholarly writing and in many airport self-help guides. Much of the literature to date regarding leadership focuses on the "how" of leading. Bohmer (2012)[2] summarizes much of the current academic research concerning medical leadership and makes a compelling argument for the "why" of leadership in medicine. In answering the question about why, we need a renewed focus on medical leadership. Bohmer (2012) has noted the growing complexity of medical care, the "professional bureaucracies" clinicians operate in, and the considerable challenges of bringing about health care reform.

Others[3-5] have argued that because of the complexity of health care delivery today, only clinical teams can impact performance improvement at the organization level and influence practice. The growing body of literature supports such thinking and confirms that good results are not a function of individual caregivers alone but also the functioning of the systems in which these individuals deliver care. [ii, iii]Collaboration among front-line staff, clinicians, and senior management is the key to changing practice and culture.

Lean Is Both a Philosophy and a Practice

It is hard to define leadership. What do we mean by "lean leadership?" Lean practice as defined by Liker and Meier (2006) in *The Toyota Way Fieldbook* stated it best for me.[6] I found myself going back to the first chapter over and over my first 3 years of working with lean. The first chapter of this beginner's lean book spells out 14 principles. *Four* principles senior leaders may struggle with the most in their first few years include the following:

First, "Base decisions on a long-term philosophy, even at the expense of short term financial goals." This one is tough, but you may have to spend some money to improve your site's quality and return on investment. Many senior leaders struggle here in that they do not have a well-articulated vision/philosophy to guide them and if they do they often feel "forced" to compromise them for the short term.

Second, "Building a culture of stopping to fix problems, to get quality right the first time." This is a frighteningly new concept in health care. Fast is encouraged rather than doing it right the first time in many health care organizations.

Third, "Growing leaders who thoroughly understand the work, live the philosophy, and teach it to others." This is tough because here we are talking about a new way. Lean is new for many in health care and even senior leaders do not know it or live it yet.

Fourth, "Go and see for yourself to thoroughly understand the situation." Simply stated, you must "know to problem solve." Many leaders do not "know" much of what goes on in areas they are in charge of. Going to the "gemba" is critical. We as senior leaders have a lot to learn about a new way to problem solve and it is uncomfortable at times.

It's About Your Staff and Customers, Not Just Bottom Lines

Many leaders fall into the trap of learning all the "tools and methods" to close gaps (cost reductions, increased productivity, etc.) and forget about the staff and patients along the way. The strength of lean is in harnessing the power of your workforce and delivering value to your customers. If their collective voices and wisdom are lost, then so is your transformation effort.

In the lean business improvement model, leaders learn that the experts needed to fix any process are the front-line staff in their organization—the "experts." This is the only way to continuously improve. Teams that have an engaged leadership can solve real problems with their customers.

Too often lean is implemented as a set of tools by a trained set of staff that "do lean." It is a tremendous developmental and organizational challenge to execute lean not in this manner but as the robust "change model" that it can be. A lean leader must be utilizing A3 thinking in all areas of their work to model this for others.

When first introducing lean to your staff, it is essential that the reasons for change be clearly communicated. Part of the process involves spending time repeatedly explaining "the what and why of lean" prior to rolling out your process improvement efforts. I recall learning the following: The first name that was given to lean was the "respect for humanity system," thus emphasizing that our goal should always be to generate value for the customer, society, and the economy; true problem solving can only be done by exploring root causes—not solving for symptoms; lean is for the scientist in all of us; a true leader does not tolerate overburdening their workforce; and if we want to keep getting better, then we must be managing for daily improvement. If we introduce lean as a "remover of waste" and introduce flow cells and concepts of pull and flow, then we will have focused on *concepts/tools* and *not people*.

Change in *culture and practice* is an incredibly difficult task—one that requires a structured approach that can be easily communicated and that engages many different levels of staff, customers, and suppliers of your health care system. For us, lean is that system; that is the strength of lean as a philosophy and practice. Often change efforts are top-down. Many smart leadership teams struggle excessively to implement powerful ideas because their key people are not engaged in the process. Lean is a change model that incorporates cultural elements and practice elements of change that can bring about true transformation if utilized as intended and done properly. Lean is not easy.

Lean is a business improvement system that starts with leadership setting the vision and ensuring all staff have what they need. Human development is the first true north metric we tackle so that the system may deliver safe quality care.

Our journey in learning and applying lean as a system for transformation began with going back to mapping our basic infrastructure so that we could then strip waste from these established processes. For the majority of our events, we first had to determine basic staffing patterns and roles to serve our patients. We had to ask ourselves if we had the right people doing the right job, when and where the patients needed them. Once that was secured, we had to review evidenced-based practices and ensure that our staff had the training and tools to deliver safe quality care. After some of these basic needs were addressed, we had to develop data systems that could help us identify quality and safety issues in real time to inform continued improvement. It is hard to strip waste from processes if processes do not exist. The lean focus on five core true north metrics took an enormous amount of energy and time to understand.

Sensei Application at Kings County Hospital Center

Not everyone at HHC has had my experience of being on rapid improvement event (RIE) teams, being a team leader, process owning, and then moving on to become a facilitator. I was in a pressure cooker job for 6 months trying to deliver some impossible results before lean was brought in to help me and my team in the CPEP. After the initial shock of all that lean entailed, a few of us realized what a unique opportunity it was to have monthly visits from a lean coach. Our team valued this kind of assistance with problem solving, and 2 years into our efforts we presented our early work at the American Psychological Association annual conference.

At the start of these insights, I discussed a colleague's tough love and fear of change. I know my friend meant to dissuade me with her article, but instead she provided me with a concise guide to process improvement for my new job that turned out to be quite accurate!

Notes

1. Chakravorty, S. (2010). "Where Process-Improvement Projects Go Wrong." *Wall Street Journal*, January 25.
2. Bohmer, R. (2012). in improving services. Harvard Business School Division of Research and The Kings Fund.
3. Melinos, J. (2001). Saving money, saving lives. In *Harvard Business Review on Turnarounds* (pp. 115–132). Cambridge, MA: Harvard Business School Publishing Corporation.
4. Abrahamson E. (2000). Change without pain. In *Harvard Business Review on Leading Through Change* (pp. 127–140). Boston: Harvard Business School Publishing Corporation.
5. Kotter, J. P. (1996). *Leading change.* Boston: Harvard Business Review Press.
6. Liker, J. K., & Meier, D. (2006). *The Toyota Way fieldbook: A practical guide for implementing Toyota's 4p's.* New York: McGraw-Hill.

Index